Michele

D1431526

The Alzheimer's Caregiver

Dealing with the Realities of Dementia

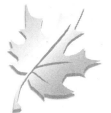

also by Harriet Hodgson

Alzheimer's: Finding the Words
A Communication Guide for Those Who Care

The Alzheimer's Caregiver

Dealing with the Realities of Dementia

Harriet Hodgson

CHRONIMED PUBLISHING

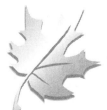

The Alzheimer's Caregiver: Dealing with the
Realities of Dementia © 1998 by Harriet Hodgson

All rights reserved. Except for brief passages for review purposes, no part of this publication may be reproduced, stored in a retrieval system, or transmitted, in any form or by any means, electronic, photocopying, recording, or otherwise, without the prior written permission of Chronimed Publishing.

Library of Congress Cataloging-in-Publication Data
The Alzheimer's caregiver / by Harriet Hodgson

     p.   cm.

Includes index.

ISBN 1-56561-125-X $12.95

Edited by: Renée M. Nicholls
Cover Design: Garborg Design Works
Text Design & Production: David Enyeart
Art/Production Manager: Claire Lewis
Printed in the United States

Published by
Chronimed Publishing
P.O. Box 59032
Minneapolis, MN 55459-0032

10   9   8   7   6   5   4   3   2   1

Notice: Consult a Health Care Professional. Because individual cases and needs vary, readers are advised to seek the guidance of a licensed physician, registered dietitian, or other health care professional before making changes in their health care regimens. This book is intended for informational purposes only and is not for use as an alternative to appropriate medical care. While every effort has been made to ensure that the information is the most current available, new research findings, being released with increasing frequency, may invalidate some data.

This one is for John,
an intuitive and kind caregiver,
a tender and loving husband.

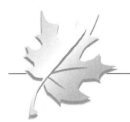

Table of Contents

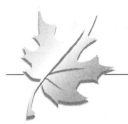

Using This Book

This book summarizes the latest Alzheimer's caregiving research. I have woven my mother's story into the research to make it come alive. In medical literature, health professionals are called "primary caregivers" and family members are called "secondary caregivers." These are misleading terms because the work family caregivers do is hardly secondary.

So these are the terms I use:

➤ *Professional caregiver* (doctors, nurses, nursing assistants, public health nurses, etc.);

➤ *Family caregiver* (adult child, niece, nephew, or other relative);

➤ *Spousal caregiver* (a special category because special problems are involved); and

➤ *Others* (friends, neighbors, other concerned people in the community).

The book will help you care for a loved one, a friend, a neighbor, a colleague, a nursing home patient, or maybe even a stranger in need. Each chapter examines a different caregiving problem and offers solutions to it. More important, each chapter ends with a summary of action steps called "What Can You Do?"

The book is aimed at caregivers in general. However, some chapters pertain to one type of caregiver more than another. For example, chapter 1 focuses on family caregivers. Chapter

6, "I Have a Boyfriend," which is about sexuality, focuses on spousal caregivers. Still, all caregivers will benefit from the research summaries and tips that are offered.

Page through the book before you start reading, to get an idea of its structure. Scan the bibliography, too, because it contains lots of leads. We're all pressed for time, but try to complete the forms in the appendixes.

Finally, remember that the caregiving you do isn't just a job; it is sacred to life itself.

Caregiving
Demands Our Best

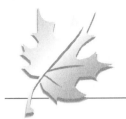

I answered the phone on the third ring. It was my mother. "I'm not moving to Minnesota!" she yelled. "It's too cold."

"But the arrangements are all made," I answered. "We've got our plane tickets and a hotel reservation, your moving date is set, and your townhouse is lovely."

"Well, I'm not moving," she repeated.

Mom had become a danger to herself, and persuading her to move to Rochester, Minnesota, had taken a year. I had to follow through, but what should I say? "You were the one who called to tell me you were found wandering in a Sears store. You said it was a scary experience."

Silence. Although I could hear Mom breathing, she didn't say anything. "Do you remember calling me?" I asked gently.

"No," Mom said.

"Well, that really happened, and you were also in a car crash. Plus, you've had several mini strokes. You need to be close to your family now."

Mom sighed a long, weary, defeated sigh. "All right, I'll come," she agreed.

I reviewed the moving plans with her again. My husband and I would fly to Florida, start packing her goods, and arrange for a tag sale. Later, we would return to Florida to finish packing, supervise loading, and drive home in my mother's car.

It turned out that we moved Mom just in time—two

more weeks and I'm convinced she would have been a bag lady.

She had been deteriorating mentally ever since my father died in 1982, when she had her first transient ischemic attack, or mini stroke.

Against the advice of family and friends, she moved from the house on Long Island where she and my father lived, to Melbourne, Florida, to be near her sister. Three years later, her sister died. Mom missed her terribly and, despite church friends and a nearby cousin, lived a solitary life.

From our phone conversations, I could tell she was getting more forgetful, using poor judgment, and spending too much money. The thrifty mother of my childhood had been replaced by an avid spender. Every phone call included a reference to a major purchase. Gold jewelry. A china cupboard. Two new cars.

A nondriver all her life, Mom managed to get her license at age seventy-nine and bought herself a new compact car. When she took the car in for its first service check, a salesman sold her a new Cougar off the showroom floor. It had leather seats, a computerized dashboard, a radio/tape player, wide racing tires, and a "hot" engine.

In addition to becoming an avid spender, Mom became an avid traveler, visiting Scotland, Italy, Greece, Alaska, and parts of America. One Saturday she called to tell me she was "out west."

"What state are you in?" I asked.

"I don't know," she said.

"Well, what town are you in?"

"I don't know."

"Where are you now?"

"Oh, I'm in a phone booth," Mom replied cheerfully. "I'm on a bus tour and having a wonderful time. We're going home tomorrow. I can't talk any more because the boat is going down the Colorado." Then she hung up.

I pictured Mom, always a woman with a zest for life, wearing a pith helmet, clinging to a rubber raft, and splashing through roiling rapids. I started to laugh and then I started to cry. Mom was a growing source of worry. What would she do next?

At Christmas time she gave my husband a light bulb —Mom thought it was a lamp. At Easter time she missed the flight from Minneapolis to Rochester and accepted a ride from a stranger. Thank goodness she called from the airport to tell me this news. I said it wasn't wise to accept a ride from a man she didn't know.

"What can he do to me?" Mom asked.

The stranger turned out to be an IBM engineer, and a genuine Good Samaritan, who recognized my mother's dementia. He drove Mom to the Rochester airport, as promised. Although the incident haunted me for months, Mom forgot it quickly. In fact, she forgot the entire trip. I didn't realize how much her mind had failed until I visited her.

I was shocked when I walked into her condominium. Newspapers, magazines, mail, and coupons covered every flat surface. Discarded shoes and clothes lay where Mom had dropped them. The air smelled of rotting garbage and the kitchen was a public health nightmare.

Mom was wearing dirty clothes—a few coffee drips here, a few ketchup drips there, and chocolate drips all down the front. Worse, her closets were crammed with new clothes, many with price tags still on them. Although Mom wore a size sixteen or eighteen, the clothes were size six or eight.

My mother had no concept of personal safety. During my visit she kept walking around nude in front of the windows. Her condominium overlooked a golf course. If I could see the golfers, they could see Mom. That didn't stop her from going "au naturel."

At night she locked the front door and put in a burglar bar.

But she left the back patio door unlocked and open, with only the screen across. To compensate for the warm, moist air, Mom turned the air conditioner thermostat to the lowest possible temperature and slept under an electric blanket.

Somehow, Mom could fix simple meals. She insisted on driving us to the grocery store. I agreed, only because I wanted to observe her driving. Several months before she had driven into the path of an oncoming car and sustained multiple injuries. Was this an isolated incident?

When I saw the car up close, I almost changed my mind. The car was so riddled with dents and scratches it looked like a battle-scarred tank. It seems Mom drove by sound —when she hit something she changed directions. Yet I was pleased with the way she fastened her seatbelt, checked the mirrors, and backed out of the parking space.

Instead of using hand-over-hand steering, Mom held the bottom of the steering wheel and inched her way around the corner with agonizing slowness. Suddenly she floored the accelerator. The Cougar raced forward with an amazing—and alarming—burst of speed. At this rate we'd pass the grocery store before Mom saw it.

But she fooled me. Mom slammed on the brakes, made a wide turn into the parking lot (narrowly missing a car), and came to a lurching stop across the white lines. "See, I can drive!" she exclaimed.

Well, I wouldn't call it driving. Mom could make a car move and that's about it. The visit convinced me I was doing the right thing. Whether she wanted to or not, it was time to move Mom to Minnesota. Getting her there proved to be the challenge I anticipated.

On moving day Mom sat in the middle of the living room. She refused to budge. This slowed down the crew and they didn't finish loading the van until 6:30 P.M. My husband and I were exhausted. We took Mom with us to the hotel and treated ourselves to a nice dinner—the only bright spot in the trip.

The next morning, when we went to get Mom from her room, she was gone. I was frantic. After searching the hallways and lobby area, we found her in the hotel restaurant. She was just about to pay for breakfast with a worthless credit card.

I'm ashamed to admit we lost her again. Later, while we were paying for gas, Mom went to an adjoining store to buy souvenirs. After that, we didn't let her out of our sight.

The trip to Minnesota took us three days. However, the moving van did not arrive for a month because of the stops it made along the way. During this time, Mom lived with us. Her stay tested my stamina.

I couldn't get a good night's sleep because Mom had a tendency to wander. During the day, she would follow me around the house, stand inches behind me, and breathe down my neck.

Since her only interests were eating, watching television, and sleeping, it was difficult to entertain her. Finally, the van reached Rochester, and we could move Mom to an assisted living community.

While Mom napped, I unpacked boxes, arranged furniture, hung up her clothes, made her bed, and stocked the kitchen. A retirement community executive came by with a welcoming bouquet. Things are working out, I told myself. Mom would enjoy our family activities and the benefits of assisted living. Besides, how hard could caregiving be?

I had a college education and lots of life experience. When I was growing up, Mom and I had been like sisters, and we could be this way again. We'd go to antique stores and craft shows and bake cookies together. Like other inexperienced people, I didn't know what awaited me.

I didn't know Mom had left a trail of debts and poor investments.

I didn't know she was the target of scams and fraud and that I'd get involved in a class-action lawsuit.

I didn't know she would become an addictive spender and write bad checks, and that I'd have to confiscate her charge cards.

I didn't know she would have more ministrokes, a massive stroke, and develop diabetes.

I didn't know she would become prone to falls, break her shoulder, and smash her face.

I didn't know she would forget she had twin boys, my father's name, and my father's death.

Most of all, I didn't know how painful it would be when Mom forgot me.

Nobody told me caregiving would be like this. Right before my eyes, my mother has been slowly dying. An accurate diagnosis of Alzheimer's can only be made after death, so I'm not sure she has the disease. However, I know she has all of the symptoms.

Maybe the diagnosis doesn't really matter. Mom is ninety-three years old, and general wear and tear on the body, as well as other illnesses, equal Alzheimer's disease. Most of the day she is vegetative, and she continues to decline. As her power of attorney, I continue to manage her finances and monitor her care.

Alzheimer's strikes older people, and more and more of them are showing signs of dementia. Forty-seven percent of the people in our country who are over age eighty-five have symptoms of Alzheimer's. The disease will be a major health problem in the years to come. Researchers are looking for early markers of Alzheimer's, ways to delay it, and ways to deal with it.

One thing is sure, being an Alzheimer's caregiver takes energy and courage. While the patient's mental abilities are decreasing, the caregiver's responsibilities are increasing. It's an inverse ratio. All of us, whether we're professional or family caregivers, ask the same question: Can I be a good caregiver and still take care of myself?

The answer is yes, but we have to work at it. Certainly, every patient deserves the highest standard of care possible. That's what we would want. For many, caregiving evolves into an ethical and spiritual journey. Caregiving demands our best and—if we let it—brings out the best in us.

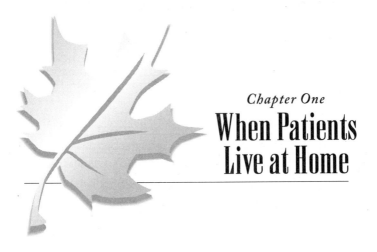

Chapter One
When Patients Live at Home

Alzheimer's disease kills brain cells. Without a functioning mind—the body's computer—the lungs stop breathing and the heart stops beating. If the patient doesn't die of other diseases first, he or she will die of Alzheimer's. Some patients live for months and others for years.

Doctors are getting better at early diagnosis. Many patients who receive an early diagnosis know what's in store for them. In her article "Living With Alzheimer's," Associated Press writer Andrea Hamilton discusses home care for such patients and stresses that "there is still plenty of living to be done." One of the caregiver's main goals is to help the patient live out life to the fullest.

It's easier to be a caregiver if you live in the same town as the patient. Long-distance caregiving is another story. The title of an article in the *Alzheimer's Association National Newsletter* states the problem clearly—"Distance Complicates Caregiving." The article says that families in this situation tend to wait for something catastrophic to happen before they make the appropriate arrangements for care.

Home care is often the best choice, especially in the early and middle stages of the disease. This kind of care has two distinct advantages: it keeps the patient in a familiar place, and it is less expensive. One half to two thirds of the people with dementia-type illnesses live at home. Of course, that home has to be a safe place.

SAFETY AT HOME

Try to see the home through the patient's eyes. Keep in mind that Alzheimer's patients perceive objects and colors differently than we do. Are the traffic patterns clear? Is the home relatively free of clutter? Will the patient have to climb stairs? Make a list of the safety hazards you find and correct them. Community agencies can help you do this. "Making Home a Safe Place," published in the *Alzheimer's Association National Newsletter* includes the following safety tips. (I have expanded the list.)

➤ Use nonskid rugs.
➤ Install safety equipment as needed (bed rails, ramps, etc.).
➤ Hire cleaning services to conserve your energy.
➤ Store harmful cleaning products in a safe place.
➤ Remove items that could be misidentified (cooking gadgets, appliances, curling irons, etc.).
➤ Put extra locks on doors to prevent wandering.
➤ Post a list of emergency numbers by the phone. If you have an automatic dial feature, enter these numbers into the system.
➤ Set the water heater temperature at 120 degrees.
➤ Remove mirrors if they upset the patient.
➤ Remove fragile and glass objects.

So-called "kiddie gates" aren't recommended by the Alzheimer's Association because they can't withstand adult weight.

Tuck electrical cords behind furniture to keep the patient from tripping. Wind long cords on special reels, available at hardware stores. Avoid extension cords, if you can, and overloading electrical circuits. A few small changes add up to big improvements in home safety.

After my mother's experience I think it's a good idea to

buy home fire extinguishers. Mom took a frosty can of soda out of the refrigerator and put it in the microwave to warm it up. The can exploded, caused a meltdown, and started a fire in the appliance. She managed to wheel the microwave cart outside without getting hurt. This time Mom was lucky, but the incident could have caused a major fire in her townhouse and adjoining homes.

Smoke detectors should be installed throughout the house. Replace any detectors that are more than nine years old, and make sure the batteries are working. It's also a good idea to install carbon monoxide detectors in the home. Review home safety regularly in light of the patient's needs.

FOOD AND BEVERAGES

Take steps to ensure food safety. The patient should wash his or her hands with antiseptic soap before eating. Alzheimer's patients often hide food in strange places, so check drawers, pockets, and purses. One day I found pieces of rotting chicken (wrapped in tissues) in Mom's purse. I found more spoiled food behind the curtains of her nursing care room.

For most of us, eating and drinking are instinctive behaviors. Not for those with Alzheimer's. The patient may lose all interest in food. Why? An article in *Day By Day: Caring For Patients With Alzheimer's*, a newsletter sponsored by Parke-Davis, explains the reasons.

According to the article, "A Little Planning Makes Eating Right A Piece of Cake," patients may forget to eat, lose their appetites, or find the food unappealing. The article offers some simple solutions:

➤ Serve familiar dishes.
➤ Serve courses one at a time (to cut down on confusion).
➤ Monitor condiments.
➤ Make sure the patient eats a balanced diet.

When you serve hot foods, make sure they're not too hot, or the patient may get burned. Also, make sure you know what the patient has eaten, because some eat other people's food or hide food in pockets and purses.

Whenever Mom came to dinner on Sunday evenings, I fixed her favorite foods—lamb chops with fresh mint sauce, mashed potatoes and rutabaga, and really good meatloaf. (There is such a thing.) Mom liked to have a glass of wine before dinner, but I was concerned; diabetics shouldn't drink wine. I talked with her doctor, who said that a small glass of wine with ice in it would be OK.

"It all comes down to the quality of life," he explained.

The Sunday dinners were a treat for Mom, and initially she thanked me for them. "Your dinner was delicious," she would say. Over time this was shortened to "Thanks for everything." This was shortened to "Thanks." Finally, she said nothing at all.

Caregivers also need to watch for signs of weight gain, weight loss, malnutrition, and depression. Be alert to self-medicating behaviors as well, such as excessive alcohol consumption. You should also inspect the contents of the refrigerator, something I learned the hard way.

The first time my husband and I went to Florida, Mom tried to serve us spoiled food. Somehow she managed to bake a dessert from scratch, a fresh plum tart with a shortbread crust. At one time the tart must have been enticing, but it had been on the kitchen counter so long a greenish-gray mold was growing on top. Mom didn't see the mold and cut a large slice for each of us.

"This food is spoiled," I said. "Do you see the mold on top? We can't eat this."

"Then I'll throw it out," Mom replied angrily, and left the kitchen. I could tell her feelings were hurt.

The next time we went to Florida I cleaned out her refrigerator in preparation for moving. It was a nasty experience. Mom hadn't covered the leftovers and the refrigerator smelled rank. I picked up a pitcher that contained a dark substance. "What's this?" I asked.

Mom peered into the pitcher intently. "I think it's gravy," she said. "Yes, it's beef gravy."

"Well, it isn't gravy any more," I answered, turning the pitcher upside down. Nothing came out. Other fossil foods had been pushed to the back of the refrigerator. The freezer was stocked with pizza and ice cream. Clearly, Mom hadn't been eating the right foods or safe foods. I'm surprised she didn't get food poisoning.

Hydration
Many Alzheimer's patients suffer from dehydration. They either forget to drink enough water or drink the wrong things. If the patient drinks caffeinated drinks, the benefits of hydration are less because caffeine is a diuretic. Remember that juice, soups, and milk count as hydrating liquids.

You might want to stock the refrigerator with ice water, carbonated drinks (without caffeine), bottled or carton juices that don't require mixing, and weak or decaffeinated tea. Iced herb teas such as raspberry and peach are a refreshing change. The idea is to make hydration easy.

MAKING A CARE PLAN
A care plan helps both patient and caregiver. Geri Richards Hall, MA, RN, CS, and her colleagues discuss care plans in their article "Standardized Care Plan: Managing Patients at Home." They think a "person-environment" should be the framework of any care plan.

According to the authors, all of the patient's behavior has meaning, and the patient has the right to be comfortable. The patient also has the right to feel like he or she has some control over things. The article includes a standard home care plan for Alzheimer's patients. The plan has three basic steps:

Step 1: Identify the problem or need.

Step 2: Identify a short-term goal to meet the problem or need.

Step 3: Identify interventions (or solutions) to help the patient.

Let's say the patient is becoming more fearful—that's the problem. The caregiver's short-term goal is to make the patient less fearful. Solutions to the problem could include looking through family photo albums and reminiscence therapy. According to the authors, a simple plan is easier to modify and adapt.

Hall's plan was originally designed for nurses, but I found it could also be used by family caregivers. Although I didn't make a formal plan, I made a list of topics that made Mom angry and led to conflict. The topics on my list included:

➤ Dismantling Mom's Florida home;
➤ Moving her to a condominium in Rochester, Minnesota;
➤ Buying what was advertised in the paper;
➤ The red coat she bought with a bad check;
➤ The deaths of friends;
➤ Moving to a studio apartment.

Over time I crossed some topics off the list and added others. I thought of ways to deal with these topics, right down to practicing dialogue. While I couldn't avoid all conflict, I could be prepared, shorten my responses, and use distraction techniques.

If you're taking care of an Alzheimer's patient at home, you need to make a care plan. Start with the basics, such as a daily routine, weekly menus, and what to do in case of emergency. The patient's doctor and public health nurses can help you work out other points. Patient exercise should be part of the plan.

Exercise

The benefits of exercise are well known. Nancy L. Mace and Peter V. Rabins, MD, co-authors of *The 36-Hour Day*, believe exercise does three things for people with dementia-type illnesses. It helps to calm them (especially agitated patients), keeps them involved, and promotes sleep at night.

Mace and Rabins point out that you might have to exercise along with the patient.

Talk with a doctor before the patient starts to exercise, especially if there is a history of heart disease, high blood pressure, or arthritis. Exercise may include stretching, chair exercises, or walking.

Walking is the best form of exercise. Usually nursing homes have railings in the hallways to help walkers. Many of the newer nursing homes have fenced gardens with landscaped walking paths. Not all caregivers have long hallways or a fenced garden, but you can walk with the patient in an enclosed mall or in your neighborhood.

The patient should wear comfortable shoes. Check the patient's feet for bunions, blisters, long toenails, and ingrown toenails. Some may need special shoes. For example, Mom's podiatrist said she shouldn't wear high heels or flat shoes, but shoes with a slightly raised heel.

Mace and Rabins think the patient should exercise at the same time each day. Short sessions are better than no exercise at all.

After exercising, the patient may want to rest. To help him or her distinguish rest time from bed time, have the patient rest in a comfortable chair or a recliner.

Medicine

To be on the safe side, store medicine in a locked cabinet. Dispose of all out-of-date prescriptions. Call the patient's doctor to make sure the prescriptions are still necessary. Are there special instructions? What are the side effects? Can the dosages be lowered?

Many elderly patients with Alzheimer's are already taking a variety of medications. A doctor prescribed sleeping pills for my mother. I got so I could tell, by the pitch of her voice and the pace of her speech, if she had taken the pills. The pills had long-lasting effects and, as Mom said, "make me dopey."

That didn't prevent her from taking them, and she began to rely on pills for sleep. After several phone calls, I convinced Mom to stop the pills and to skip daytime naps. I also started keeping a list of her medications. The list helps me help Mom.

If you're a long-distance caregiver, arrange for someone to monitor the patient's medications. Call a public health nurse, a reliable neighbor, or a church friend. Other geriatric services may be available in the area, so check the local phone book. You want to make sure the patient is taking the right medicine in the right way. Unfortunately, many patients don't do this.

Geriatrician Eric Tangalos, MD, of the Mayo Clinic's Alzheimer's Disease Center, says half of the patients who leave his office fail to take their prescriptions or they take them improperly. Often times, the elderly (including those with dementia) reduce the prescribed dosage to "save money" or because they're confused. Doctors call this practice self-rationing. Self-medicating is just the opposite. The person prescribes over-the-counter medicine for himself or herself or takes medicine on hand to feel better. These people may also take more than the prescribed dosage to feel better faster. Both practices are dangerous. "Educating people and keeping them healthy through prescription drug compliance makes good sense medically and financially," Dr. Tangalos writes in the *Rochester Post-Bulletin*.

My mother's insurer, Minnesota Comprehensive Health,

provides me with regular reports on the prescriptions that have been filled for her. The local pharmacist also provides me with reports, including which nonprescription medicine she receives. I keep these reports in a special file. They're helpful at tax time and for tracking purposes.

Driving Issue

Driving is a thorny issue for caregivers. Bring up the topic, and family members will tell you a story about a loved one getting lost, a near-miss, or a horrendous accident. Certainly, Mom's driving sparked terror in me.

It increased when I heard some of her stories.

Once, she got on the wrong highway, left the Melbourne city limits, and headed for Louisiana. Another time she drove through a deluge of rain. "It rained so hard I couldn't see the road," Mom began. "You know, in Florida you have to turn on your lights when it rains. I turned on the car lights, but I couldn't see anything."

"Did you pull over?" I asked.

"No, I just kept going," Mom replied. "It took me two hours to get home."

What worried me most was Mom's total lack of concern. In her mind there was nothing wrong with driving a car when you couldn't see. From her earlier description, I figured Mom was several blocks from her condominium when the storm hit. She must have been driving around in circles. Thank goodness she got home safely.

I think chance is the crux of the driving issue. Will this be the day the patient's mind loses more data? Sense of direction? Coordination? Reaction time? Judgment?

Driving will continue to be an issue in the years ahead, especially as the population ages.

Licensing. Many patients in the early stages of Alzheimer's continue to drive. Are they safe? Richard M. Dubinsky, MD, and his colleagues examine the issue in their paper

"Driving in Alzheimer's Disease." The authors surveyed sixty-seven patients from the Alzheimer's Disease Clinic at Kansas University Medical Center and compared them with one hundred elderly controls. Survey questions included such topics as driving habits, why they stopped driving, how they were affected by weather and time of day, speed, and accidents. After a statistical analysis of data, the authors concluded that driving should be a careful consideration for Alzheimer's patients and that relatives should keep them from driving, if necessary.

"Removing driving privileges requires an objective and reliable method of identifying unsafe drivers prior to an accident," the authors say. But how can we evaluate these drivers safely? Dr. Dubinsky and his colleagues are considering the use of something called an "interactive computer-based simulator."

Harold N. Mozar, MD, and James T. Howard, MS, of the Alzheimer's Disease Program at the California Department of Health Services, also discuss driving in a letter to the *Journal of the American Neurological Association*. They point out that California uses three criteria to determine a driver's competency: medical data, a personal interview, and testing under controlled conditions when necessary.

I don't think Mom would have passed another driver's test, not after getting five speeding tickets and being court-ordered to a refresher course. My cousin showed Mom how to get to the course. However, she couldn't find the address again—a test in itself—and never took it.

Years ago, she had started taking driving lessons. The lessons were going well until Mom drove into the front porch. When my brother and I heard the thud, we knew just what had happened. Through the porch windows, we could see the impaled car, its fender crunched on the corner of the porch, and Mom behind the wheel looking slightly dazed.

My brother, who had a quick wit, opened the front door and called, "Did you knock?" I knew he was trying to diffuse the situation with humor. It didn't work. Mom lost what little confidence she had gained and didn't complete the course.

To get a license at age seventy-nine was a major achievement for her. She managed to get her license by good coaching and lots of driving practice. Mom had reason to be proud. Yet I had reason to be fearful. Just before we left Florida, I arranged to have her license revoked. Unfortunately, losing her license not only took away her independence, it also took away some of her self-esteem. Denial was her solution. Mom continued to believe she had a license in her wallet and enjoyed telling stories that began, "When I'm driving..."

Bathroom Issues

Using a bathroom and going to the bathroom are difficult tasks for Alzheimer's patients. Caregivers need to make sure the bathroom is a safe place. Use rubber-backed bath mats to prevent the patient from slipping. Put nonskid strips on the tub and shower.

Make sure the bathroom is well lit. Mom liked to have a night-light in her bathroom. She also kept a flashlight by her bed in case the power failed. I think these are good ideas.

Many accidents occur when patients are stepping out of the tub or shower. You might want to buy a shower bench and install a grab bar next to the tub. The grab bar should be fastened to the wall studs. Buy a free-standing toilet seat if the patient has difficulty using the toilet.

As my mother's dementia got worse, it became harder for her to stand. She would lurch sharply from one side to the other when walking and couldn't get out of a chair without help. We were going to put a grab bar in the bathroom and buy a special toilet seat, but time ran out. Mom's mental abilities took a dive. Our sweet Sunday dinners became so frightening we had to cancel them.

Elimination. The time comes when the patient can't tell if he or she has to go to the bathroom. Accidents happen. The patient may get to the bathroom too early or too late. Patients in the later stages of the disease become incontinent. This can be a major concern for home caregivers. First, you need a large supply of protective garments such as Depends. Second, the cost of these garments adds up quickly. Third, caring for an incontinent patient is time-consuming and unpleasant.

Try to keep the home odor-free. Discard protective garments in a trash can with a tight-fitting lid to cut down on odors. Remember to look around the house (under beds, chairs, and in cupboards) for discarded protective garments and soiled underwear. Dispose of trash quickly.

Many patients, particularly women, develop bladder infections. Caregivers need to be aware of the symptoms of infection: a continuous urge to void, painful voiding, and chills. If you think the patient has a bladder infection, call his or her doctor immediately.

Using Support Services

I keep hearing stories about spouses who don't have the physical strength to take care of patients. One husband nearly dropped his wife while trying to get her out of the bathtub. The family caregiver may think home care is no longer possible. However, with the help of outside services, home care may continue for a while longer.

Don't be ashamed to ask for help. You have to take care of yourself in order to care for someone else. There are many support services available. Call your local Alzheimer's Association and ask for a pamphlet called "Alzheimer's

Disease: Support Services You May Need." Other helpful resources are:

➤ The Alzheimer's Association (national and local);
➤ Your county health department;
➤ The Salvation Army (which may offer adult day care);
➤ Senior citizens groups;
➤ An area Council on Aging;
➤ The Eldercare Locator, U.S. Administration on Aging.

Colleges and universities are also responding to care-givers' needs. Amy Anderson, EdD, RN, nursing chair at Regis College in Weston, Massachusetts and her colleagues came up with a plan to help nursing students care for Alzheimer's patients and their caregivers. They detail the plan in an article called "Unsung Heroes."

The plan is based on five main points: Problem Identification, Assessment, Creative Problem Solving, Emphasis, and Simplicity (PACES).

Care problems were sorted into seven groups. Group one included diagnosis and characteristics of the disease. Group two included behavior and mood problems. Group three covered the many problems of daily care. Group four covered health problems. Group five focused on caregivers' problems. Group six dealt with the legal aspects of care. And group seven included respite and nursing home care.

Thirty-one learning units were developed for the nursing students. The students did not provide initial advice to the caregivers; first, the caregivers told the students what they needed, such as bereavement care. The students then suggested solutions to the caregivers.

The training plan worked so well Anderson and her colleagues think the modules may eventually be used with family caregivers.

"It is the caregiving families who are the unsung heroes of community-based Alzheimer's care," they write. "Our goal is to recognize them and to assist them in this arduous task."

Countering Loneliness

Progressive dementia leads to loneliness. If you can't remember your daughter's visit, you're going to be lonely.

If you can't remember how to socialize, you're going to be lonely. If you can't remember your family, you're going to be really lonely. Before long, the patient will withdraw into his or her own world.

There are ways to counter loneliness. Some caregivers set up regular visiting schedules. To help the patient remember their visits, family members and friends sign a guest book.

Pet therapy has become popular, so popular that some nursing homes have a resident pet. If you've ever watched someone with Alzheimer's cuddle a puppy, you know why. The residents of my mother's retirement community take turns walking a dog. Mom loved it. "He was a big dog, like the one you have," she said. "I didn't walk him; he walked me!"

Adult day care is another way to counter loneliness. The programs are geared especially for Alzheimer's patients. Activities range from music therapy to crafts. While the patient is at day care, the caregiver gets a much needed break.

Anya Lockert describes yet another way to counter loneliness in her article "Finding Comfort in Rituals." She describes a program at the Huger Mercy Living Center in Phoenix, Arizona. Priests who have Alzheimer's disease live together in a cottage at the center. Despite memory problems, the priests remember how to say mass, and find comfort in the ritual. Mass brings them together and is a way to counter loneliness.

Many nursing homes schedule regular visits from school

children. The residents perk up immediately when the children arrive. Nothing seems to counter loneliness like children's voices. That's why I connected our twin grandchildren with Mom as often as possible. "They're darling," Mom would say. "Just darling."

HANDLING INCREASING NEEDS

Memory loss is an early sign of Alzheimer's, and it gets progressively worse. The patient is unlearning. Some experts think a home environment helps to prolong the patient's self-care skills. In the medical literature, these skills are called ADL, Activities of Daily Living. Unfortunately, the patient's ADL skills decline steadily.

Leslie Jean Neal, MS, RNC, CRRN, CS, discusses self-care skills in her article "The Home Care Client with Alzheimer's Disease: Part 1." According to Neal, patients lose the ability to perform sequential tasks, such as driving before they lose the ability to perform self-care tasks, such as bathing. She suspects this is because the basic skills are learned in childhood.

While observation is most useful, Neal thinks assessment tools are helpful in measuring ADL abilities. She recommends the Blessed Dementia Rating Scale and the Instrumental Activities of Daily Living Scale, developed at Duke University. "Other scales may not transition well into the home setting," she writes.

Neal also thinks home health care nurses need to become familiar with assessment tools. Family caregivers do, too. For more information on mental assessment tools, contact a physician or a neuropsychologist.

No matter how well we plan, the time comes when home care isn't enough. Professional care is needed. The decision to put a loved one in a nursing home is gut-wrenching and painful. Family members may feel guilty about the decision. But deep down inside, they may also feel relieved.

Is It Time for a Nursing Home?

I was relieved after Mom moved into the assisted living community. As much as we loved her, having her with us for a month taught us a valuable lesson: she couldn't be a permanent resident. My husband and I were so tired we could hardly get our work done.

There was also the safety factor to consider. We lived in the country, and there were no street lights. Unless there was a full moon, the night sky was pitch-black, and you could hardly see anything. Mom could wander outside and get lost or fall.

Fortunately, I found a marvelous retirement community for her, with townhouses, apartments, and studio apartments. All had assisted living services. Before a resident moved in, the apartment was painted and carpeted, and new drapes were installed. The monthly fee covered cleaning, linens, dinner, electric bills, heat/air conditioning, TV hookup, and an activities program. Other services were available on a fee-for-service basis.

If a resident hadn't been seen, a staff person would call to check on that resident. The retirement community also had a nursing care wing, a feature that turned out to be crucial for our family. Putting Mom in nursing care is one of the most painful decisions I've ever made. How do you know when this time has come?

"When It's Time to Consider Other Options," an article in the newsletter *Day By Day: Caring For Patients With Alzheimer's,* a service of Parke-Davis, asks caregivers to answer some key questions. I have expanded the questions and added some of my own:

➤ Has home caregiving become too much for you to handle?

➤ Do you think the patient is safe in your home?

➤ If other family members live with you, how are they handling home care?

➤ Can the patient still perform basic self-care tasks?
➤ Are you using any support services?
➤ Is your stress level going up?
➤ Do you take the time to take care of yourself?
➤ Have you lost control of your life?
➤ How does the thought of professional care make you feel?
➤ What is the financial impact of caregiving on your family?

You may think of other questions as well. It may take a while, but the answers to these questions will come to mind. The patient's safety is the deciding factor. Ask yourself, "What's best for the patient?" Then do the right thing. Sadly, Alzheimer's may impede the patient's understanding of your motives and actions.

The Patient's Fear of Abandonment

I had discussed nursing care transfer with Mom. "You don't want me any more," she replied. In the midst of winter, when the wind chill factor was seventy-six degrees below zero, she threatened to run away. Would she do it? If Mom fell in the snow, she could easily freeze to death.

Worried and scared, I called her doctor at home. "It's time, Harriet," he said. "Your mother has to go to nursing care. I'll write special admittance orders for her."

I told Mom she had so many health problems that she needed professional care. For Mom, one of her worst fears had come true; she thought we had abandoned her.

Hanns G. Pieper, PhD, discusses the fear of abandonment in his book *The Nursing Home Primer: A Comprehensive Guide to Nursing Homes and Other Long-Term Care Options*. He thinks the fear comes from the false idea that older people are dumped in nursing homes, only to be forgotten by family. "The fact that this stereotype does not reflect reality does not reduce the fear felt by many persons at a time when their whole world seems to be going haywire," he explains.

The Impact on a Marriage

Alzheimer's not only affects the parent-child relationship, it has a devastating impact on a marriage. Researcher Lore K. Wright, at the Medical University of South Carolina, studied thirty couples and published his findings in *Social Science & Medicine*. In each instance, one spouse had been diagnosed with probable Alzheimer's disease, and the other was the primary caregiver. The couples were referred by one of seven agencies and were interviewed at home.

According to Wright, a slow interview pace was used, and cue cards were used with the Alzheimer's patients. The mean age of the caregivers was 67.4 years. Twenty-four of the primary caregivers were female, and six were male. This group was compared to a group of seventeen "relatively healthy" couples. Wright was honest about the limitations of his study: the small statistical sample, nonrandom subjects, and two-year data collection time.

Still, one of his findings is worth noting. Wright discovered that the patient's educational level had a lot to do with nursing home placement. Highly educated patients moved out of their homes and into nursing homes sooner than less-educated patients. Why? "One possible explanation is that declining capacities of highly educated afflicted spouses make the contrast between what *was* and what *is* more hopeless for caregiver spouses." In short, the spousal caregiver lost hope.

Perhaps nursing home placement was a way of facing loss, Wright speculates, or the caregiver may have had the financial means to pay for professional care.

SUMMARY

Home care continues to be a growing trend for three reasons. First, there's a shortage of nursing homes, and many have waiting lists. Second, the family may think the patient is too old to move. Finally, experts say that cost is the main reason families choose home care. "A primary goal in caring for these clients is to keep them at home for as long as possible because an estimated $13 billion is spent annually on in-home care," writes Leslie Jean Neal, "compared with an approximate $41 billion spent for nursing home care."

All across this nation, in bustling cities and sleepy towns, family members are caring for Alzheimer's patients at home. It can be a hard, lonely road. The journey is easier if you take some of the following action steps.

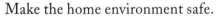

What Can You Do?

Make the home environment safe.

Take steps to ensure food safety.

Watch for signs of weight gain, weight loss, malnutrition, and depression.

Work out a simple home care plan.

Store medicine in a locked cabinet.

Monitor prescription and over-the-counter medications.

Keep the patient from driving, if necessary.

Use available support services.

Counter loneliness with appropriate activities.

Use mental assessment tools.

Prepare for the patient's feeling of abandonment. Ask yourself, "What's best for the patient?"

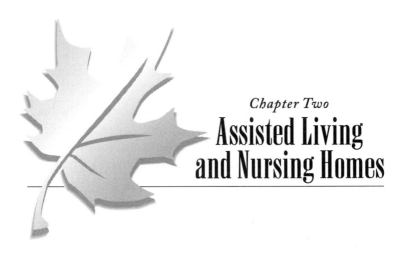

Chapter Two
Assisted Living and Nursing Homes

Assisted living gives the Alzheimer's patient a safe place to live while maintaining some control over life. This kind of living has many pluses. An article in *Assisted Living Today,* "Marketing That Pays," lists some of the factors to consider in choosing an assisted living home:

➤ The range of services (covered by a monthly fee)
➤ The location of the facility (close to family)
➤ The rates (residents get a lot for their money)
➤ The resident's previous address
➤ The trained staff and available support services
➤ Hospital/religious affiliations.

Kensington Cottages in the Midwest provide assisted living for people with memory problems. There are Kensington Cottages in Buffalo, Mankato, and Rochester, Minnesota; as well as in Bismark, North Dakota; and in Waterloo, Iowa. The cottages are homey. "Our focus is on a social model of care, rather than a medical model," says Briana Melom, Family and Education Coordinator in Rochester.

Each cottage has four apartments, which are located at the corners of the building, with common space in the middle. Caregivers receive eight hours of Alzheimer's training. Although the caregivers do the cooking and laundry, residents are encouraged to help out. The activities program also includes many daily living tasks.

Keep in mind that assisted living isn't necessarily long-term residence. Some residents are there only a few months. "When you know one Alzheimer's patient, you don't know them all," Melom says. "Each patient is different, so we can't predict a general length of stay."

What are some of the discharge factors? Kensington Cottages has four main criteria:

➤ Are two caregivers needed to help the resident walk?
➤ Does the resident need twenty-four-hour skilled nursing care?
➤ Is the resident immobile or bedridden?
➤ Has the resident become a serious threat to others?

Melom thinks the time may come when Kensington Cottages offers nursing care. Rochester is the fastest growing location for Kensington Cottages and more may be built in the future. This approach fills a growing need for people with dementia. Similar facilities are popping up in other parts of the country. In the next section, I discuss how to find them.

FINDING AN ASSISTED LIVING FACILITY

Look in the yellow pages of the phone book and start calling. Ask for written information, a sample activities schedule, a fee schedule, and admittance criteria. If you know people who have a loved one in an assisted living facility, talk with them. Are they satisfied? Does the resident seem satisfied? Would they change anything?

Visit each facility that interests you and pay special attention to:

➤ General atmosphere. Is it attractive and suited to the residents' needs?
➤ Attitudes. Do the residents seem comfortable and interested in life?

➤ Supervision. What is the staff-resident ratio and is there adequate supervision?

➤ Exercise. Is there a place for the residents to exercise and walk?

➤ Activities. Are the residents involved in appropriate activities, such as gardening?

➤ Standards. Does the facility meet public health standards?

➤ Inspection. Is the facility inspected on a regular basis?

➤ Individual needs. Does the staff respond to the residents' needs and treat them with dignity?

Give yourself some thinking time. Study the information you've received and visit each facility again. You want to find the best possible match for the patient. To be on the safe side, also start looking at nursing homes now. Put the patient's name on a waiting list, if necessary.

When Mom moved into a retirement community with assisted living services, I was relieved. Here she could be independent and protected at the same time. Socializing with a cross-section of people was another advantage of the community. Mom enjoyed bus trips, luncheons, concerts, and more. That all changed when she went to nursing care.

NURSING HOMES

Seth B. Goldsmith, author of *Choosing a Nursing Home,* says the facilities fall into three general types: skilled nursing, intermediate care, and residential care. The classification indicates the kinds of services that are offered. He writes, "While the definitions of the various levels are ambiguous, the states also issue detailed regulations about requirements in terms of specific services and staffing for each level."

Finding the right nursing home can be confusing. It can also be time-consuming. According to Goldsmith, there are vast differences between nursing homes. The nursing home may be government-owned, not-for-profit, or private, and each may have a different philosophy. There are other variables to consider, too, such as staff training, quality of activities, and management.

Special Care Units

An increasing number of nursing homes have a Special Care Unit for Alzheimer's patients. Dorothy B. Smith is Assistant Professor at Northwestern Louisiana State University in Shreveport. Her article "Staffing and Managing Special Care Units for Alzheimer's Patients" discusses these units.

Smith thinks having a Special Care Unit requires some special management decisions. These decisions include a carefully screened staff, indoctrination, staff support/continuity, and Alzheimer's education. Staff members should be the kind of people who are really interested in the patients' lives—past and present. As Smith points out, the Special Care Unit is the patient's home. She recommends the use of special clothing or symbols (a patch or a pin) to promote staff unity. The staff should receive the support it needs, a sense of job security, and Alzheimer's training.

"Nursing assistants should be trained to learn communication skills that will enable them to work with the family and include them in the patient's care," she writes. Smith is convinced that one person can make a huge difference in the patient's care.

George Washington University Medical Center conducted a national survey of Special Care Units. For years, nobody was sure what the Special Care Units standards should be. Even now, standards are evolving as more is learned about Alzheimer's. The survey had two purposes: to develop a "snapshot" of the units and to establish a baseline for studying trends. Joel Leon, MD, summarizes the survey in his article, "The 1990–1991 National Survey of

Special Care Units in Nursing Homes." Leon points out that Special Care Units differ in design; some are self-contained and others are a clustering of patients.

Licensed nursing homes were surveyed by a self-administered questionnaire. Thirty-five percent of the 15,555 eligible facilities didn't respond. A statistical analysis of data turned up an interesting finding. Only 9.6 percent of the 15,555 licensed facilities had Special Care Units. Does the patient need a Special Care Unit or will he or she do just as well in a general nursing home?

Making a Choice

The choice may hinge upon what is available. Before you choose a nursing home, Leon says, there are many things to consider:

➤ Security (limited access off and on unit).
➤ Design (individual/communal space, square footage, circular hallways, etc.).
➤ Special dining and activity areas.
➤ Reduced environmental stimulation.
➤ Admission criteria.
➤ Staff ratio and training.
➤ Special activities for residents/families.

A U.S. Department of Health and Human Services publication, *Guide to Choosing a Nursing Home,* tells more about nursing home standards. The booklet, which is available at your local Social Security office, ends with a three-page nursing home checklist. How do you make the choice? For me, medical care and safety were the deciding factors. I could not provide the medical care and ongoing monitoring that Mom needed.

If the patient is going to share a room, try to find a compatible, friendly roommate. Also, find out how much furniture the patient may bring from home. My mother has a swivel chair, a chest of drawers, and a nightstand.

Interior Design. Frank Mahnke, president of the International Association of Colour Consultants, says nursing homes should avoid disturbing colors such as red or black. Soothing colors such as rose should be used instead. Alzheimer's patients may think large animal prints are alive, so these should be avoided. Small patterns should be selected for fabrics instead.

Recently the nursing care unit of Mom's retirement community was renovated. All of the above recommendations were followed. Brown carpeting was replaced with rose and teal carpet squares that could be replaced easily. Brass chandeliers were hung over the dining room tables. A photo name plate was put on the door of each resident's room. New artwork was hung on the walls, along with a list of the goals of nursing care. The nursing station was angled to make it more accessible, and a separate meeting room was created from existing space. This room, which is opposite the nursing station, is used for craft activities and worship services.

It was clear that a lot of thought had gone into the renovation, and I was delighted with the results. Although Mom watched the work in progress, she didn't seem to understand what was happening. Still, I think she benefited from the renovation in many ways.

Soothing Places and Spaces. Nursing homes are responding to the patients' needs in other ways. John Hendren describes a unique approach in his article "In 'Snoezelin Room' Alzheimer's Takes a Nap." (Snoezelin is a combination of the Dutch words for sniffing and dozing.) He tells about a new addition to a Baltimore nursing home, a room that combines rest with sensory stimulation.

The room is like an artist's blank canvas. A curtain of fiber-optic tubes changes color. A wind machine blows gentle breezes, and a water tower makes bubbling sounds. Patients hear wind chimes and songbirds, and sometimes pictures are projected on the walls. Staff members think the room calms patients without the use of drugs.

As more is learned about Alzheimer's, caregivers know patients need to be connected with nature. Without this connection, their lives become even more insular. Something as simple as a window box filled with red geraniums and trailing vines can bring great pleasure to patients who find it interesting to watch flowers bud and bloom and change. A bird feeder in a tree can provide endless hours of enjoyment.

Soothing places and spaces like these also connect the patient with changing weather and seasons. These are important connections because they help the patient keep track of time. Seasonal activities help as well.

Activities. Despite their disease, Alzheimer's patients can enjoy a variety of activities. The activities may be links to the past, such as playing catch, singing familiar songs, or painting. In some cases, the patient's activity and occupation are the same.

Artist Willem De Kooning was diagnosed with Alzheimer's in 1989. He continued to work, painting nine-foot square canvases on exhibit at the Walker Art Center in Minneapolis. Mary Abbe discusses the exhibit in an article called "Walker Exhibit Examines Final Works of De Kooning, Art Giant with Alzheimer's."

She thinks the show is about the man. Experts disagree on when the artist started losing control of his mental abilities. Art critics wonder about the impact of Alzheimer's on his work. Other experts think the disease may have spared his procedural memory. "De Kooning might have been able to go on painting long after he ceased to understand why," Abbe explains.

Mom's nursing home offers a variety of activities—exercise, trivia time, scout visits, cooking experiences, concerts, choral groups, sing-alongs, manicures, bingo, and stories read aloud. When I was a child, Mom loved books. As her reading ability faded, having someone read to her became more pleasurable. After she lost the ability to process incoming sound, she stopped going to story time.

BEHAVIOR PROBLEMS IN NURSING HOMES
Wandering

Research shows that living in a nursing home may contribute to such behavior problems as wandering, agitation, sundowning, shadowing, and combativeness. Dr. Taher Zandi discusses behavior problems in his article, "Understanding Difficult Behaviors of Nursing Home Residents: A Prerequisite for Sensitive Clinical Assessment and Care." Dr. Zandi thinks wandering may a symptom of the instinctive desire to search for home, "to recapture the feelings of safety and belonging."

Certainly, Mom wanted to turn back the clock and live on Long Island. Sometimes she thought she was there. I had seen other residents wandering about, but never thought Mom would join them. She was one of the smartest people I'd ever known. For several months her dementia stayed the same—it plateaued—and then took a dive.

Mom started to wander. She was living on Nursing Care East and would walk to the Nursing Care West wing. After she moved to the Nursing Care West wing, she walked back to Nursing Care East. I think she needed somewhere to go. She would peek in a door, shake her head, and say, "No, not there." What was she doing?

One day Mom said, "When my husband comes to get me (she couldn't remember his name), we'll have to find a place to live." I told her Dad had died more than twelve years ago.

Instead of upsetting her, my answer seemed to comfort her. "Oh, that's it," she said. "I've been looking for him and looking for him. I couldn't find him anywhere."

A wave of grief washed over me. I wanted to cry for them both, for my father, whose name she couldn't remember, and for my mother, who searched for him diligently. Maybe that's why Mom was wandering. Other experts think wandering is caused by a highly active lifestyle in the past. All I know is that Mom's wandering got worse.

Agitation

Wandering is a sign of agitation. Linda A. Gerdner, MA, RN, and Kathleen C. Buckwalter, PhD, RN, FAAN, discuss this behavior in their article "A Nursing Challenge: Assessment and Management of Agitation in Alzheimer's Patients." They define agitation as having three components: aggressive behavior, such as kicking another nursing home resident; physical nonaggressive behavior, such as nudity; and verbally agitated behavior, such as repetitive phrases.

Agitation affects the patient's general health. In fact, the authors report that it has led to more falls. "Research also has found a relationship between sleep and levels of agitation," they write. These disruptions may lead to altered biological rhythms.

Too much stimulation—television, PA systems, crowds, loud music, conversation, testing fire alarms, and the like—can cause agitation. Sensory impairment may also contribute to agitation. Pain, parkinsonism, heart problems, electrolyte disturbances, and endocrine disorders may all lead to agitation. Finally, drug toxicity may produce agitation. After reviewing the literature already written on the subject, Gerdner and Buckwalter recommend:

➤ Creating a controlled environment that allows pacing (circular hallways, a safe outdoor area);

➤ Keeping a daily routine (to make the patient feel more secure);
➤ Checking the patient's physical condition;
➤ Serving balanced meals (smaller portions, finger foods, adequate liquids);
➤ Getting new glasses and hearing aids when necessary.
➤ Breaking down tasks into smaller steps;
➤ Using nonthreatening body language and gestures;
➤ Simplifying the environment;
➤ Using helpful therapies (music, tactile stimulation, reading aloud, doll play).

Despite all of these possible solutions, the authors say agitation is still a pervasive problem. Taking care of an agitated patient is a challenge for any caregiver. Two other behaviors, sundowning and shadowing, may also challenge our caregiving skills. Let's take a look at these behaviors and their causes.

Sundowning

Sundowning is defined as late afternoon or early evening agitation. The symptoms include restlessness, panic, confusion, and angry behavior and language. Dr. Taher Zandi, of the Northeastern New York Alzheimer's Disease Assistance Center, says, "There is no explanation for why some persons 'sundown' and others do not."

The causes of sundowning are unclear. It may be caused by less light, fatigue, boredom, and stress. What's more, the patient's biological clock may be off. Other medical problems may also contribute to sundowning.

Improved lighting may help to decrease the patient's wandering. Daily exercise also helps the patient get rid of some nervous energy. Snacks may help to divert the patient, and experts recommend cutting back on caffeine. Simplifying the patient's environment also has a calming affect. Some patients have been helped by doll and pet therapy.

You may think of more solutions. Sundowning can be difficult for home caregivers to handle because they're fixing meals at that time. To make matters worse, sundowning may be combined with shadowing.

Shadowing

No, this isn't a weather forecast; it's rather scary behavior. Shadowing is defined as following closely behind another person, imitating them, or both. I admit that Mom's shadowing made me nervous. When I took a step, she took a step. If I turned to get something out of the refrigerator, I'd bump into her. She kept this up for hours at a time.

While she was shadowing me, Mom was also criticizing me. I spent too much time cleaning. Living out in the country wasn't a good idea. That outfit looked awful on me. The house was too cold or too hot.

Patients who are shadowing others may be emotionally fragile. All caregivers need to approach these patients slowly. Speak in a gentle voice. Focus your remarks on the patient's feelings. You might say, "It looks like you're worried about something." Use short sentences and avoid getting into an argument with the patient.

Remember, this isn't deliberate behavior; it is the result of Alzheimer's disease. Shadowing may be as uncomfortable for patients as it is for caregivers. Maybe more so. The patient's agitation continues to build as the disease progresses. Before long agitation may also give way to combativeness.

Combativeness

Combative behavior is the result of frustration. The causes include sensory overload, misunderstanding things, and differentiation problems. In short, the patient can't cope. An Alzheimer's Association fact sheet, "Combativeness," in the program notes for the third Mayo Alzheimer's Disease Center Conference for Families, "The individual may feel that he's being pushed to do something that simply can't be done." In that case, the caregiver should step in. For example, if the patient can't get his or her arm through a sleeve, the caregiver should perform the task.

Combative patients should be monitored carefully. Overly aggressive behavior may warrant transfer to another facility. However, there are things we can do to help the patient before this happens.

Dr. Zandi recommends cutting back on demands. We can also validate the patient's feelings. Look for things that may contribute to the patient's behavior, and avoid or remove them. Finally, give the patient emotional support through gentle words, touches, and expressions. "Anticipate and avoid agitation," he summarizes.

MENTAL ILLNESS AND NURSING CARE

Alzheimer's disease is listed in the *Diagnostic and Statistical Manual of Mental Disorders (DSM)*. This means the disease may cause mental illness. Cynthia Steele, RN, MPH, and her colleagues examine psychiatric problems in their article "Psychiatric Symptoms in Nursing Home Placement of Patients with Alzheimer's Disease." Two-hundred ten patients with possible or probable Alzheimer's were involved in the study. The patients were examined by a psychiatrist. They were interviewed and given neurological and mental examinations. The researchers examined twenty-five patients after nursing home admittance.

One predictable finding: Nursing home patients had more problems with self-care. The nursing home patients also had more behavior problems and were more depressed. "We found that potentially reversible psychiatric symptoms such as depression and agitation were among the important predictors of nursing home placement," the researchers explain. Mental problems may be evidenced by delusions and hallucinations.

Delusions

Delusions are beliefs that are contrary to the facts. British researcher Alistair Burns and colleagues focused on mental problems in their paper "Psychiatric Phenomena in Alzheimer's Disease." Burns conducted one of the few studies that combined interviews, mental assessment tests, and computerized tomography (CT) scans.

A total of 178 Alzheimer's patients were involved in the study. The researchers found a lower number of delusions in patients than in previous studies, and two results caught my attention. A sizable number of the study participants had delusions of persecution. Men were more apt to have delusions of theft.

I'd seen Mom's CT scan, which was riddled with holes, and I didn't need photos to tell me she had cognitive deficits. References to delusions were woven into her daily conversation. Her biggest delusion was that my father was going to rescue her from the nursing home. This delusion continued until she became vegetative.

Mom also believed my brother, who had been divorced for years and had remarried, was going to marry his first wife again. A long and involved story was invented to go with the delusion. The story was pure confabulation, a blend of fact and fantasy, and she told it often.

Delusions can be frightening for Alzheimer's patients. One elderly female patient was being wheeled into the bathroom for her morning bath. Sensing the patient's hesitancy, the caregiver chatted about how nice the bath would feel. But the patient thought she was being taken to a strange place to be killed.

"I don't want to die! I don't want to die! I don't want to die!" she screamed. "Don't take me in there."

Since I witnessed this incident, I've read more about delusions. Evidently, the sound of running water upsets many patients. The patient may not recognize a bathroom or its uses. If you didn't know what a bathtub was, wouldn't it look strange to you?

Hallucinations

The Dictionary of Psychology defines a hallucination as a "false perception; the acceptance of ideational phenomena as real." Hallucinations can be very frightening for Alzheimer's patients because they are so real. I'm not sure when Mom's hallucinations started, but I know she had them in her studio apartment. They seemed to increase when she went to nursing care.

One hallucination involved a flock of birds. We were standing in front of her bedroom window when she told me the story. "I was awake in the middle of the night," Mom said. "When I'm awake I look outside at the moon. There wasn't a moon last night." She paused a moment, as if she were seeing the scene again.

"A flock of birds came and landed outside my window. They were big black birds."

"I don't think many birds fly at night," I replied, regretting the words as soon as I voiced them.

"Well, they were there. The birds landed on the grass and they stayed there all night. There were lots of them, dozens and dozens. I think they were crows. In the morning, when I looked out, they were gone."

The conversation made me wonder about Mom's other hallucinations and how often she had them. At least the bird hallucination was harmless. What about the other hallucinations, the ones that scared her or caused night terrors? Mom's failing language skills prevented her from telling any more about hallucinations. I wonder what secrets are locked in her mind.

Lowering Stress. Caregivers can help hallucinating patients. One of the first things we can do is lower the patient's stress. Noise is a major stressor for patients. During the renovation described earlier, one patient sat up suddenly and yelled, "Quiet! Quiet! You _____ of _____! If there's a lady or gentlemen here, I would pay you to keep quiet!" Her head fell forward, and she looked like she was asleep until she added, "And I would pay you well!"

Music, however, may help to lower stress. Mary Sambandham, MSN, RN, and Victoria Schirm, PhD, RN, discuss music in their article "Music as a Nursing Home Intervention for Residents with Alzheimer's Disease in Long-Term Care." While the patients listened to music, researchers observed their reactions and evaluated them with a music therapy assessment test. The patients talked less while listening to music and seemed to be more alert afterward. The researchers also believe that music cued memories and helped the patients to express their feelings.

COMMUNICATING WITH PATIENTS

If we're going to communicate with patients, we have to fine-tune our communication skills. Caregivers may need special training. One training program is detailed in "Alzheimer's Disease Caregivers: The FOCUSED Program," by Danielle N. Ripich, PhD and her colleagues. Their article was published in *Geriatric Nursing.*

Chair of the Communications Department at Case Western Reserve University, Ripich designed a communication skills program for caregivers. To help caregivers remember the seven communication steps Ripich uses the acronym FOCUSED. What do the letters represent?

F stands for face-to-face communication.

O stands for orientation, another way of saying repeating.

C stands for continuity—the caregiver signals topic changes.

U stands for helping patients become "unstuck" by providing words for them.

S stands for structure, giving patients a choice from preselected options.

E stands for exchange, the basis of all communication.

D stands for direct, short sentences and gestures the patient can understand.

All of these tips are good ones, but the **U** tip, providing words, didn't work for me. Mom became angry when I filled in blanks for her or finished sentences. My "helpfulness" emphasized her conversational helplessness. I found it was better to let conversation lapse, than to point out Mom's verbal problems. Still, the FOCUSED acronym reminds caregivers of these communication tips.

Caregivers may also derive satisfaction from improving communication. Judith M. Richter and her colleagues studied how family members communicated with fearful, agitated, and wandering patients, and the researchers presented their finds in their paper "Communicating with Persons with Alzheimer's Disease: Experiences of Family and Formal Caregivers." Two kinds of caregivers participated in the qualitative study: formal (or professional) and family. The purpose of the study was to compare communication techniques and processes. Twenty-three family caregivers were contrasted with twenty-two professional caregivers (nursing assistants). Data was collected in focus groups.

The caregivers discovered two common themes: environmental adjustments and reassurance. Family caregivers who communicated with fearful, agitated, and wandering patients took practical steps to improve the setting, such as cutting down on noise and closing the blinds. They reassured patients by staying close to home and sticking to a routine.

Professional caregivers adjusted the environment by locking doors and removing the patient from the scene. Some of the nursing assistants were frustrated by their efforts to communicate. One is quoted as saying, "Evenings are the worst…there's no way to reach them then."

According to the researchers, family caregivers felt more helpless than the professionals. The researchers say many family and professional caregivers don't have sufficient communication training, and "the turnover of nursing home staff compounds this problem." They see a need for more training and recommend tailoring communication techniques to the patient. A team approach is also recommended.

CARE CONFERENCES

Care conferences are a way for nursing home staff to meet with the patient's family and to coordinate patient care. Care conferences also foster the team approach. The state of Minnesota requires nursing homes to conduct care conferences every three months. Written notification of the conference date is sent to the family. After the conference, a family member signs a form to prove it took place.

At Mom's care conferences, I bring up topics that are bothering me. Sometimes the professional caregivers have a different slant on things than I do. At one conference a new staff member told me she had a "nice conversation" with my mother.

"Please don't say that," I said, knowing Mom was vegetative most of the time. "Her doctor thinks she has lost the ability to process incoming sound, and she understands very few words."

But the staff person stuck to her story. I promised to visit Mom after the conference was over. The conference went quickly because there wasn't much to say about Mom.

She was on a liquid diet, losing weight, and bewildered.

Mom was almost asleep when I went to see her. To get her attention, I grasped her hand. "You hand is cold," she said.

Hmmm, maybe I had been wrong. Maybe the staff person did converse with her. Certainly, she spent more time with Mom than I did. On the other hand, she didn't know Mom as well as I did. "Well, it's chilly out," I replied. Mom said, "T-6, B-2," and pulled back her hand. Anything else she said was bingo talk, a jumble of letters and numbers. She was still talking bingo talk when I walked out the door. The sounds still rattle around in my head and I can't get rid of them.

HOSPICE CARE

Alzheimer's patients in the final stage of the disease may benefit from hospice care. "Families Find Comfort in Hospice Care," an article in the *Alzheimer's Association National Newsletter*, discusses the advantages of a hospice. The article says "Hospice (also known as palliative care) programs—typically associated with cancer and AIDS—focus on comfort and care."

Working closely with patients, the hospice staff strives to keep patients free from pain and to understand their concerns; the staff also counsels family members. The patient doesn't necessarily have to move into a hospice. Many communities offer hospice services to home-bound patients via public health programs. Currently, there are eighteen hundred hospice programs in the United States. Call the National Hospice Organization at 1-800-658-8898 for more information.

TROLLING FOR DOLLARS

New products and services have been created to meet the growing needs of patients. Some business people have been less than ethical in an attempt to get new clients. Take the case of Herman, who had lived in a nursing home for four years. In addition to Alzheimer's disease, Herman had high blood pressure, had suffered some ministrokes, and then had a massive stroke.

Herman was hospitalized a week and returned to the nursing home. By now the stroke damage to his brain was substantial. That didn't stop a speech therapist from calling his son. "I think I can help your father," she said. "With speech therapy, I think he could speak more clearly."

"Although my father rarely speaks—he's had so many strokes, the words he says are clear," the son replied. "My father doesn't need speech therapy; he needs a new brain."

As the speech therapist continued her sales pitch, the son realized she wasn't familiar with his father's medical history. She was trolling for dollars. The son refused speech therapy again. What happened? The speech therapist reported him to the authorities for mistreating a vulnerable adult. Fortunately, the son had been a good caregiver and the report was thrown out.

I'm sorry to say this isn't an isolated incident. There are vultures out there, waiting to snatch funds and goods. In one case, when family members went to get their mother's personal effects after she died, they discovered the painting over her bed had been stolen. It was never found. Jewelry and clothing have been stolen from other nursing home patients.

Many catalogs have been published that feature Alzheimer's products, such as expensive speech kits. It's true that speech kits can help to stimulate speech, but you could probably make your own kit for less. Better yet, you can tailor the kit to the patient.

Most caregivers are selfless, dedicated people with the patient's welfare at heart. We can only admire their courage. Despite all of the problems—hallucinations, delusions, shadowing, sundowning, agitation, wandering, and adjusting to group living—they continue to help the patient. Here are some of the action steps you can take.

What Can You Do?

Research assisted living facilities and nursing homes.

Find a nursing home with a Special Care Unit if you think it's necessary.

Find the best match for the patient.

Create soothing places and spaces.

Involve the patient in appropriate activities.

View wandering as the instinctive search for home.

Take steps to curtail agitation.

Be patient with sundowning and shadowing.

Be alert to psychiatric problems and get professional help, if necessary.

Take steps to improve communication.

Participate in care conferences.

Bypass inappropriate therapies and services.

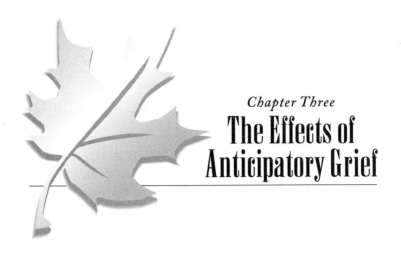

Chapter Three

The Effects of
Anticipatory Grief

Anticipatory grief is a controversial subject. Some experts think you can't grieve for something that hasn't happened. Other experts think anticipatory grief is real and powerful. Lack of definition, poor research, and conflicting studies fuel the controversy. What is anticipatory grief?

DEFINITION

Anticipatory grief is mourning before death has taken place. Therese A. Rando, PhD, a psychologist in Warwick, Rhode Island, is an expert on this kind of grief. She discusses its complexities in her article, "Anticipatory Grief: The Term Is a Misnomer but the Phenomenon Exists."

"Just because anticipatory grief is not exactly like post-death grief…does not mean it is not grief," she writes.

According to Rando, anticipatory grief is a response to past, present, and future losses. I certainly think a lot about life without a mother. Mom has spent a lot of time thinking about life without a husband and friends. At age ninety-three, she has outlived almost all of her friends, and lives in a world filled with strangers.

Some experts think anticipatory grief is an instinctive response. Dr. Robert Buckman explains the response in his book *"I Don't Know What to Say": How to Help and Support Someone Who Is Dying.* He says, "We grieve before a death just as we flinch when we anticipate being injured." Thinking about a loved one dying of Alzheimer's disease can cause

41

caregivers to flinch, but some caregivers deny this grief and its subprocesses.

ANTICIPATORY GRIEF SUBPROCESSES

The rising number of Alzheimer's cases may be sparking anticipatory grief research. Much of this research is on the structure of grief. Therese A. Rando reports on four overlapping subprocesses of anticipatory grief in her book *Loss & Anticipatory Grief*:

➤ Awareness (coming to terms with loss).
➤ Affective (experiencing/coping with feelings).
➤ Cognitive (concern for the patient).
➤ Planning for the future (without a loved one).

Rando says anticipatory grief evolves over time and can be conscious or unconscious. Once the patient dies, anticipatory grief becomes post-death grief.

STAGES OF GRIEF

Like post-death grief, anticipatory grief may be divided into stages. The time you spend in each stage depends on dozens of variables. Psychiatrist Elisabeth Kubler-Ross, MD, identified five stages of grief: denial, anger, bargaining, depression, and acceptance. Caregivers may go through one or more of these stages. While the stages help us come to terms with the finality of Alzheimer's disease, each stage is a challenge in itself.

As Kubler-Ross points out in her book *On Death and Dying*, "Death is still a fearful, frightening happening, and the fear of death is a universal fear even if we think we have mastered it on many levels." We can only come to terms with death as best we can.

RESPONSES TO ANTICIPATORY GRIEF

Robert Fulton, PhD, and Robert Bendiksen, PhD, discuss responses to anticipatory grief in their book *Death & Identity*. They identified three main responses: reaction, disorganization, and reorientation—another word for recovery. While we're responding to anticipatory grief, we're also caring for the patient. We can get so busy we're hardly aware of anything.

Therese A. Rando thinks the extent of anticipatory grief depends on a variety of psychological, social, and physiological factors. Psychological factors include things such as unfinished business between the patient and caregiver. Social factors include things such as the caregiver's support system. Physiological factors include things such as the caregiver's health. Anticipatory grief is a process, Rando says, and "not an all-or-nothing thing."

OTHER GRIEF FACETS

Anticipatory grief has many facets. Oftentimes anticipatory grief is tempered with hope. "This is one of the subtle differences that makes anticipatory grief unique," Fulton and Bendiksen write in *Death & Identity*. I don't think this is a subtle difference; I think it's a startling difference. Hope and grief are opposite emotions.

If the patient is diagnosed early, caregivers may experience anticipatory grief for years. A recent Alzheimer's Association publication reported that patients are living as long as twenty years with the disease. This is a big chunk out of our lives. To complicate matters even more, anticipatory grief may start before we notice it.

Roller Coaster Emotions

Family caregivers, in particular, may experience many different emotions in a day. Our feelings may change from hour to hour. "This roller coaster effect inhibits the grieving process by aiding in what might be called denial," note co-authors Fulton and Bendiksen. "The reality of the situation is that the death is expected, but exactly when it will take place is not known."

Deep in our hearts we know that Alzheimer's is a fatal

disease, and statistics prove it. A recent issue of *American Medical News* reports that 16,754 people died from the disease in 1993. The article also says that whites are two times more likely to die of the disease than blacks. Men are slightly more susceptible to Alzheimer's disease than women.

For many family caregivers, anticipatory grief is a constant companion. According to Rando, family members may grieve for "losses yet to come," another facet of anticipatory grief. I know what she means. Although Mom is breathing, she isn't really alive. The funny, bright, articulate, kind, and eager woman I knew is gone. I grieve for the empty seat at the dinner table, the Christmas gifts I won't buy, and Mother's Day without her.

Much of what I am today is due to my mother's influence. She nurtured my creativeness as I traveled from kindergarten to college and beyond. All through life, Mom has been my primary role model and I miss her already. Death will be the final punctuation mark in a long life, a challenging life, a life well-lived. Although I believe this, I don't know how I'll respond when she dies.

Decathexis

Anticipatory grief can create problems for patients and caregivers alike. Some caregivers withdraw from the patient prematurely, a process called decathexis. Even if we know we're doing this, we may not be able to stop ourselves. As Dr. Robert Buckman explains in "I Don't Know What to Say," the grieving person may feel guilty for "having mentally buried" the still-living patient.

A caregiver who withdraws too soon may blame the patient for causing so much work and putting family members through turmoil. Anger may become part of the detachment process. "There does not have to be detachment from the dying patient prior to death," Rando writes.

The patient needs our care, concern, and love *now*. As caregivers, we have the option of staying close to the patient, respecting life for what it is, and savoring the days that remain. I've tried to do this with my mother. There are few days left and those are numbered. Still, I can feel myself detaching from her, and this makes me sad.

Systematic Decathexis

Another facet of anticipatory grief is something called systematic decathexis. This is a conscious process that involves planning for a life without the patient—a recovery plan, if you will. Eliott Rosen thinks this process has some advantages. In his book *Families Facing Death*, Rosen writes, "Systematic decathexis is reflected in the family's ability to conceive of itself as an emotionally intact unit without the presence of the patient."

Family members may consolidate the patient's financial records. The family may decide to move to a smaller location to cut down on care costs. Members of the extended family may come for a visit. Doing these things helps caregivers and patients alike.

Resurrection-of-the-Dead Syndrome

Many caregivers experience the "Resurrection-of-the-Dead Syndrome," although they may not know it. Charles David describes the syndrome in an article by the same name, and notes that the syndrome occurs when the patient is seriously ill or has survived a near-fatal accident "due to heroic intervention of medical technology, or the availability of a new therapeutic procedure."

I went through this. My husband and I attended a convention in Los Angeles. No sooner had we arrived when the phone rang. It was a hospital emergency room physician. Mom had suffered a massive stroke and was in serious condition. The doctor said he would keep me posted, and we agreed that no unnecessary measures would be taken.

I was fine until my husband left for meetings and I was alone. Immediately I started crying. "God speed, Mom," I said. "God speed."

During the day I found myself bursting into tears without any warning. Mom had signed a living will, and I had made arrangements with the funeral home. Flying the "red eye" home wouldn't do anything for Mom because she no longer knew us. My husband and I decided to stay at the meeting.

Although I expected Mom's doctor to call at any moment with the news of her death, Mom rallied. When the doctor called, he said Mom had improved so much she would be dismissed in two days. Medical technology and expert care had resurrected her from the dead. Just when I thought I'd gotten my anticipatory grief under control, it started anew.

Anticipatory grief is an uncomfortable feeling, to say the least—a feeling that sucks energy from you. After several months of emotional spadework I spoke at an Alzheimer's Association conference. I had professional slides to go along with my talk, and because I wanted to put a face on the disease, the first slide was of Mom.

The talk ended with a quote of hers that I included in my book, *Alzheimer's: Finding the Words, A Communication Guide for Those Who Care.* "Just think of the changes I've seen. When I was a child, I went to school in a horse-drawn carriage. When I was an adult, I saw men walk on the moon. I think I've lived my life at the best time."

Seeing the quote on the screen brought tears to my eyes. I really started crying when I read it. Why was I crying so? First of all, I could picture Mom going to school in a black horse-drawn carriage. I, too, had seen men walk on the moon. But it was the last sentence that really got to me. Mom had summarized her philosophy of life in one sentence.

"These words continue to inspire me," I said in a faltering voice. "Instead of moaning and groaning about things, what if we got up with the idea that we were living our lives at the best time? What could be accomplish? What changes could we spark? What wrongs could we right?"

With tears trickling down my face, I finished the talk. I scanned the audience and continued to make eye contact. Nearly everyone in the audience was crying. Alzheimer's disease had more than a face; it had a name, the name of my mother, Mabel Clifton Weil. The audience shared my grief for the woman she had been.

GRIEF TRIGGERS

The problem with anticipatory grief is that you never know what will set it off. Anticipatory grief is especially hard to handle if you're a professional caregiver and a family caregiver. Pamela N. Enlow, MSN, RN, discusses this dual relationship in an article called, "Coping with Anticipatory Grief." She talks about her mother's living death from cancer and her own anticipatory grief. "It is a morbid grief that persists with great tenacity."

Every time I thought I was calm, something else would trigger my grief. Some examples:

➤ **Facial changes.** My mother had thrown out more than $3,000 worth of goods: eye glasses, her hearing aid, and two sets of dentures. Her funds were almost gone and we couldn't keep replacing these things. Without dentures, Mom's face and profile look very different.

➤ **Family photos.** We usually take photos at family gatherings. I always look forward to seeing the developed pictures. When I see the blank look on Mom's face, however, I start grieving. Will this photo be the last?

➤ **Lack of social graces.** Mom lost the ability to use a knife and fork, although she still uses a spoon. In the past Mom had been a fastidious woman, and seeing her eat with her fingers made me sad. Sometimes she threw food.

➤ **Forgetting she had twins.** One of the greatest tragedies in Mom's life was the death of one of her identical twin boys two days after birth. She carried this knot of grief with her throughout life. The day came when Mom forgot she had twin boys and thought she had fraternal twins like our grandchildren.

➤ **Loss of reading ability.** For months Mom tried to cover up the fact that she couldn't read. Her excuse: "I don't like to read any more." This from a mother who insisted on having her own newspaper subscription in nursing care.

➤ **Loss of writing ability.** One day I found two pieces of paper beside Mom's bed. I recognized her handwriting, but the words she wrote made no sense at all. On one of the papers she had written, "Again for again. Come to aboard again love." On the other she had written, "O come to...We love for that...paid—to bed." Mom had lost the ability to write meaningful sentences.

➤ **Anger and hostility.** Mom spent all of her cash, and her investments were a mess. To conserve funds, I put her on a limited budget and approved or disapproved purchases. Like other Alzheimer's patients, Mom decided I was stealing from her. "You've got my car, you've got my furniture, you've got my dishes, you've got my money!" she screamed. "What more do you want?" I wanted to cry.

➤ **Care category.** The state of Minnesota evaluates patients on an ongoing basis and determines their care category. Care ranges from A, the least care required, to K, the most care needed. Recently Mom's category was changed to J. She doesn't have far to go.

➤ **Living will.** Mom wanted to sign a living will, and I witnessed her signature in the presence of nursing home staff. "I don't want anything!" she exclaimed. "No wires. No tubes. No reviving. None of that stuff. When I'm gone, I'm gone."

➤ **Visiting the mortuary.** Before we left on a trip, I made arrangements with a local mortuary to pick up Mom's body when she dies. Making the arrangements really triggered my anticipatory grief.

What are your grief triggers? Use the log form in Appendix A to track them. You can write the month only, if you wish. The date is important because it gives you a reference point. I would list the first grief trigger on the form like this:

Date	Incident	Why am I grieving?
Jan. 1996	Mom threw out her second set of dentures	She doesn't look like Mom.

Become aware of the ways you handle your anticipatory grief. Denial. Humor. Manic behavior. It won't do you any good to try to escape grief with frantic activity. You'll only wear yourself out. Also become aware of how long you've been grieving. Do you think you're making progress?

HOW PROFESSIONALS HANDLE GRIEF

Professional caregivers aren't immune from anticipatory grief. However, they are trained to focus on the patient's medical care and they learn how to detach from anticipatory grief in positive ways. Pamela N. Enlow refers to this process in her article "Coping with Anticipatory Grief." She says detachment is more than pulling back from the patient; it's redirecting energy "toward more productive activities."

I wanted to talk with someone who had practical experience, so I called Joan Gregor, RN, former director of nursing at Mom's nursing home. "How do you keep from crossing the line and grieving too much for the patients?" I asked. "Those people came first," she replied. "But it's because I wasn't related to them that I could take care of them."

Gregor also scheduled some decompression time. For her, this time was the drive to and from work. "I didn't turn on the radio or anything," she said. "It was quiet." And she learned how to leave her work at work. "I realized that I couldn't take everybody home with me. I had to be able to walk out the door."

But some medical professionals handle grief with denial. One patient, Pam, had lived in a nursing home for three years. One day the director of the nursing home called Pam's daughter. "I think your mother has pneumonia. She's coughing and coughing and needs to go to urgent care," she said. "We'll have her ready and the paperwork you need."

The doctor confirmed the diagnosis of pneumonia and returned the paperwork directly to the daughter. She was shocked. Despite Pam's severe dementia, under the "cognition" heading, a member of the nursing home staff had checked "confused at times." Under the "agitation" heading, "occasionally" had been checked. And under the "wandering" heading, "never" had been checked.

Pam was far worse than these ratings indicated. "I think there's a little denial going on here," her daughter said. The doctor nodded his head in agreement. Clearly, the patient in front of him wasn't the patient that was described on the form. Although it may be unconscious, denial is still denial.

THE PATIENT'S SELF-GRIEF

Patients in the early stages of Alzheimer's may experience self-grief. Why me? Why now? What will become of my family? A prominent neurologist was diagnosed early with the disease and ended his practice immediately. He wrote to his patients, explained his illness, and referred them to other physicians. He handled his self-grief with action.

The patient may grieve for things he or she did in the past and can't do now, such as playing bridge. My mother grieved for the healthy body and energy of her youth.

She also grieved for the emotional resilience she used to have. "You can adjust when you're young," she said. "It's harder to do when you're old."

Mom thought about death a lot. At first, she said things such as "When I die, you'll have to ship my body back to Long Island." A year later she was saying, "You don't have to ship my body to Long Island. Bury me anywhere. Pick a nice green spot. I don't care." From other comments she made, I concluded Mom had made peace with death.

"HOARDING GRIEF"

Americans don't like to talk about death. In fact, we hardly say the word and talk all around it. Instead of saying "died," we say the patient has passed away, bought the farm, is pushing up daisies, went to meet his or her maker, or kicked the bucket. Mom kept telling me it was time for her to "check out."

Avoiding grief only makes things worse. Bettyclare Moffatt, the author of *Soulwork,* thinks crisis, change, and responsibility can make us hoard our grief. She writes, "To keep ourselves from exploding, from falling apart, from dissolving, from dying, sometimes we hoard. We hoard our pain. We swallow our rage."

Facing anticipatory grief is a wiser approach. But before you can do that, you need to have an idea of the extent of your grief. Evaluating anticipatory grief takes some time; however, it's time well spent.

EVALUATING THE GRIEF YOU FEEL

Researchers have come up with several ways to measure anticipatory grief, including rating scales, graphs, and interviews. The interview technique may be the easiest of the three. Talk with a sibling or a trusted friend about your anticipatory grief. If you don't have anyone to talk to, try talking to yourself. This sounds silly, but Kelly Osmont, the author of *More Than Surviving*, says it works. "Others have found that just talking aloud or into a tape recorder was helpful. Some stand in front of their mirror and talk."

We shouldn't worry about doing these things, Osmont says, because we're intelligent people. I talk to myself all the time. It's a good way to try out words and sentence flow. After Mom became severely demented, I found myself talking aloud more often. The technique helps me to figure out my feelings.

Maybe you're a visual person, not a verbal person. Instead of talking to yourself, you might want to picture your grief in some way. John W. James and Frank Cherry tell how to make a loss history graph in their resource *The Grief Recovery Handbook*. They recommend this pencil exercise for post-death grief, but it helped me understand my anticipatory grief. Here are their instructions:

➤ Find a partner to help you and schedule a meeting with him or her.

➤ Don't make the graph more than twenty-four hours before the scheduled meeting with your partner.

➤ Don't talk while you're doing the graph.

➤ Get a large piece of paper and work horizontally.

➤ Draw a line across the center of the page and divide it into four equal parts. The entire line represents your age; the midpoint represents half your age; and so on.

➤ Think about your losses for an hour, and position them on the graph. Use a longer vertical line to show the intensity of the event.

➤ Study the graph and figure out its implications.

I made my graph differently. First, I folded the paper twice to make the lines. Next, instead of graphing my entire life, I graphed the last six years, which had been particularly stressful. Here's my graph.

Loss History Graph

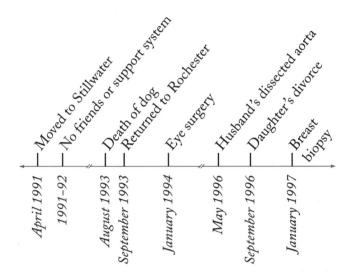

You can see the causes of my grief.

➤ Moving from our house in the country (I had supervised the construction of our dream house).

➤ Having no friends or support network in a new community.

➤ The death of our dog Max (my constant companion).

➤ Returning to Rochester and leaving another dream house (I had supervised construction again).

➤ Unexpected laser surgery for a detaching retina.

➤ My husband's dissected aorta—a real medical crisis (detailed later).

➤ Our daughter's divorce and its effects on our twin grandchildren.

➤ A recent and scary breast biopsy

Use the form in Appendix B to create your own graph. Chances are, your graph is similar to mine. Maybe now you can see why caregivers wear out. Life doesn't send us problems one at a time; they often come in bunches. I've had several "grief clusters" in my life. Chapter 9, "How Personal Issues Affect Caregiving," contains more information on this topic.

There's another way to evaluate anticipatory grief. Susan K. Theut, MD, MPH, and her colleagues used a scale method to study anticipatory grief. They explain their study in "Caregiver's Anticipatory Grief in Dementia: A Pilot Study." The purpose of the study was to evaluate a new anticipatory grief scale. Twenty-seven spouses who were taking care of patients with dementia completed the scale.

Questions on the scale covered such things as emotional closeness to the spouse, the ability to move ahead with life, the caregiver's adjustment to illness, and planning for the future. Not only did the study confirm the existence of anticipatory grief in family caregivers, it revealed other problems. The authors say anticipatory grief "extends over time and lacks closure" and see a need for more caregiver support. "Recognition of anticipatory grief as a significant factor in the spouse/caregiver's adjustment should be an integral part of such support."

Depending on what else is going on in your life, it may take you a while to process anticipatory grief. Finding ways of coping may take you longer as well. No matter how small it may be, each step brings you closer to your goal—getting through this. You can do it. Trial and error will teach you how to cope.

Coping

Edward Truschke, president and chief operating officer of the Alzheimer's Association, says the disease is increasing but continues to be underreported. More people will need to cope with anticipatory grief. The coping methods that work for one caregiver may not work for another. You'll figure out what works best for you. Consider these ways of coping.

➤ Learn about anticipatory grief.
➤ Get help. Talk with a grief counselor, a psychologist, a psychiatrist, or a member of the clergy.
➤ Let yourself cry in public and in private.
➤ Pace yourself. (I only visit Mom every seven to ten days now.)
➤ Divide tasks into smaller parts.
➤ Learn meditation and relaxation techniques.

Harriet B. Braiker suggests another coping strategy, making a pleasurable activities list, in her book *Getting Up When You're Feeling Down.* She writes, "The important thing is that you (a) know what kinds of things give you pleasure; and (b) that you do at least five pleasurable activities per week, even more if possible." The form in Appendix C will help you start your list. Do some of the things on the list afterward.

My pleasurable activities list contains some pretty quiet stuff—reading for pleasure, and going to the movies. Recently, I wanted to see a new comedy that had just been released. When the movie came to Rochester, my husband was out of town. I went to the movie by myself, and I had a good time. Laughter really is good medicine.

How Anticipatory Grief Can Help

Many experts believe anticipatory grief helps you. Edward Myers writes about prolonged death in his book *When Parents Die: A Guide for Adults.* He explains, "Weeks, months, or years of warning can give you a chance to accept the forthcoming death, to make sense of it."

In her article "Anticipatory Grief Reactions in Family Members of Adult Patients," Deborah Welch, RN, MSN, says this grief response may be an emotional rehearsal. Anticipatory grief may lessen the post-death grieving process. The anticipatory grief I felt made me more aware of life.

At this point, Mom is vegetative—her eyes are either closed or blank—yet I derive pleasure from seeing her face. I want to do all I can for her and have worked hard to manage her investments. It seems I'm moving beyond death and becoming more aware of her life as a whole.

Anticipatory grief can be a wake-up call for caregivers. We can help the patient tie up loose ends, such as making a living will and disposing of possessions. Mom wanted to give her furniture to our older daughter (the twins' mother), and she received pleasure from this.

Finally, anticipatory grief may push us in new, positive directions. According to Robert Fulton, PhD, and Robert Bendiksen, PhD, anticipatory grief helps us to accept reality. We become more comfortable with ourselves—with who we are and what we can do. "This may entail the rejection of some now unrealistic goals," they write. "It may mean a reassessment of one's life."

What Can You Do?

Read about anticipatory grief.

Become aware of the stages of anticipatory grief.

Monitor your anticipatory grief responses.

Become aware of the facets of anticipatory grief: hope, roller coaster emotions, decathexis, systematic decathexis, Resurrection-of-the-Dead Syndrome.

Keep a list of your grief triggers.

Detach from the patient in positive ways.

Think of anticipatory grief as part of life.

Watch for signs of self-grief in the patient.

Evaluate the anticipatory grief you feel.

Identify ways of coping.

List the things that give you pleasure and do them.

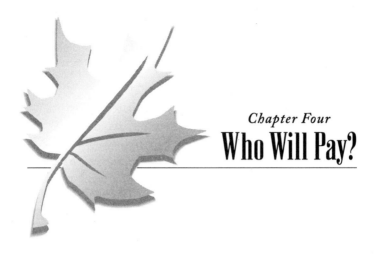

Who Will Pay?

Alzheimer's care costs are going up and many caregivers feel like they are chasing a moving financial target. You wouldn't be the first caregiver to ask, "Who will pay?" H. Gilbert Welch, MD, MPH, and colleagues focus on dollars and cents in their article "The Cost of Institutional Care in Alzheimer's Disease." They studied two hundred patients with probable Alzheimer's disease.

The patients were at least sixty years old, had exhibited the symptoms of dementia for at least three months, and were willing to be interviewed. Family members were also interviewed because patients may give misleading or false information. According to the researchers, nursing home costs are rising because of need (more Alzheimer's patients), length of stay, and "a relatively high disease prevalence."

The researchers predict that the elderly population will grow 40 percent in the next thirty years. Moreover, some 40 percent of the Alzheimer's patients will be in nursing homes "at any given time." Predictions on the number of future cases was recently revised. Some experts think the patient count will double. If the patient count continues to rise, future generations will be faced with higher care costs.

WHY ARE COSTS RISING?

Richard L. Ernst, PhD, and Joel W. Hay, PhD, analyze published cost data in their paper "The U.S. Economic and

Social Costs of Alzheimer's Disease Revisited." They identify several key reasons for spiking care costs.

First, some Alzheimer's patients are in mental hospitals, and treatment is more costly than general health care. Diagnostic costs are also rising. Alzheimer's patients use hospitals more than the general population. And finally, there are the costs of drugs, transportation, and visits by healthcare workers. "For home dwelling patients, most of this burden—nearly $31,000 per person in 1991—is borne directly by caregivers, but much of the cost of institutionalization falls on the public at large," note the researchers.

ALZHEIMER'S AND FINANCES

Many family caregivers fear bankruptcy. Alzheimer's strikes their loved ones when they have kids in college, added work responsibilities, and health problems of their own. Then too, Alzheimer's patients have been the target of scams, fraud, bait-and-switch schemes, and overpricing. It's almost impossible to retrieve these lost funds.

Patients in the early stage of disease may not realize they're in financial trouble until it's too late. That's what happened to my mother. Despite her ability to add columns of figures in her head, Mom forgot the first rule of economics: watch your cash flow. She didn't know how much money was coming in or how much was going out.

I didn't know she was low on funds until we packed her goods for moving. Not only was her bank account almost empty, but Mom had also been doing lots of impulse buying. She bought a diamond ring that cost one thousand dollars, subscribed to about ten magazines, and joined a recipe club. In addition, she was playing the lottery and, as near as I could figure out, was spending about fifty dollars a month on tickets.

"You can't play the lottery any more," I said.

Mom looked at me defiantly and shouted, "I'm going to

play the lottery!" She got a faraway look in her eyes and a pained expression came across her face. "You see, I lost some money and I'm trying to win it back."

"No more lotteries, Mom," I answered. "You don't have the money."

Several minutes later Mom walked to the door with an envelope in her hand. "What's that?" I asked.

"Nothing," she said, hiding the envelope behind her back.

I reached for the envelope and it was just as I feared, another lottery form. "It's my money," Mom said. "I can spend it the way I want!"

"Your money is gone and Dad's money is gone," I answered. "There's nothing in your bank account." Mom stared at me in surprise. However, I think our surprise exceeded hers.

My husband and I found a trail of unpaid bills, poor investments, and unpaid taxes. Her checkbook was a picture of financial and mental ruin. Between entries for power and garbage services there were entries to "prize" centers. The centers had clever names that used words such as *disbursement*, *guaranteed*, and *payout*. Sure, the checks were small, but the dollars added up.

Schemes and Scams

The phone calls Mom received also helped to explain her financial losses. One call confirmed her new subscription to *Lottery Magazine*. I canceled it. Another call confirmed her order of a hospital bed. I canceled it.

I also found a life insurance policy with my maiden name on it. "Why did you buy this?" I asked. "You already have life insurance."

"The salesman said it would be a nice thing to do for my daughter," explained Mom. I could hear the salesperson's build-up in my mind and his final pitch. And there were more plot twists in Mom's financial tragedy.

She had paid hundreds of dollars for a water filtration system that sold for less than fifty dollars in Minnesota. When she bought the new Cougar, she lost somewhere between twenty and twenty-two thousand dollars. Thousands of dollars had been invested in failed mortgages and, to make matters worse, her mind was failing when she tried to retrieve her losses. The money didn't dribble away: a hundred and fifty thousand dollars. gushed away in a flood of spending and poor judgment.

Shortly after Mom moved to Florida, she had another ministroke. The stroke damaged the part of her brain that controlled bladder function. One of the world's experts on bladder control and repair at the Mayo Clinic saw Mom and said nothing could be done. She forgot her Mayo Clinic physical, found a Florida doctor who was willing to perform bladder surgery, and called to say she was thinking about having it the following week.

"Don't have bladder surgery!" I exclaimed. "It will cost a lot of money and won't do you any good. Your problem is in the brain, not the bladder." After some hard and fast talking I convinced Mom to forego surgery.

Alzheimer's patients don't have the cognitive ability to spot scams. At a time of life when they should be wary, many are too trusting, giving people money and goods. If Mom liked someone, she would give them anything: a book, her new washbasket, a mirror off the wall. Maybe this was her way of reaching out to people in her loneliness.

COST OF CARE

Dorothy P. Rice, who is affiliated with the Institute for Health and Aging at the University of California, and her colleagues studied care costs. Their paper "The Economic Burden of Alzheimer's Disease Care" describes their study of patients in five northern California counties. Despite the study's limitations— its lack of random sample and its limited geographic area—one conclusion is worth noting.

"Informal care costs (grooming, bathing, etc.) are almost three times the cost of formal care for persons with Alzheimer's disease in the community," say the researchers. Their findings also showed that 60 percent of the services, whether formal or informal, were paid out of pocket.

Paying for these services can become a tracking nightmare. If you lack documentation, which is what happened to me, tracking is even more difficult. I bought special file cabinets for my mother's paperwork. Her documents are filed by year, and the folders are labeled Health Insurance, Investments, Life Insurance, Medical and Dental Bills, Prescription Drugs, Receipts, Social Security, and Income Taxes. To help me budget, I sat down and figured out her basic costs.

Monthly Costs

Nursing Home: Roughly $4,500 (and going up)

Prescriptions: $60–90 (and going up)

Medical Insurance: About $200 (and going up)

Other costs included nonprescription drugs, church contributions, clothing, postage, and medical and dental bills not covered by insurance. These costs add up to hundreds and thousands of dollars. Every three months I transfer funds from her cash management account into her checking account. The transfers are getting larger.

Unexpected Costs

Family caregivers have lots of unexpected costs. Transportation is one of them. Once, while we were on vacation, Mom became ill in nursing care and was sent to the hospital. Although our community has a bus for physically challenged people, it wasn't running at that time. The nursing home staff hired a companion to take Mom to the Mayo

Medical Center. The companion's fee plus the cost of the cab came to one hundred twenty-five dollars.

The bill upset me. Please understand that I'm not criticizing the companion's concern or dedication. Cab fare was a necessary expense, but a Mayo Clinic escort could have taken Mom to her appointment. Because of the companion, Mom didn't use escort services. In my mind, it cost one hundred twenty-five dollars to transport Mom less than three miles. Still, this cost is small when compared to the costs other caregivers have.

One long-distance caregiver flew to New England to visit her mother. When she arrived at the nursing home a staff member criticized the daughter for not visiting her mother more often. The comment was unnecessary and unkind. "I'm sorry," the daughter replied. "But air fare is expensive, and I can only afford to visit my mother three times a year."

The Costs of Special Care Units

Which costs more, a general nursing home or a nursing home with a Special Care Unit (SCU)? One study shows that the cost is about the same. David R. Mehr, MD, MS, and Brant E. Fries, PhD, compared costs in their study "Resource Use on Alzheimer's Special Care Units."

They studied data from 177 nursing homes in six states. Patients in nursing care units were compared to patients in Special Care Units. The data base included demographics, diagnoses, activities, cognitive performance, physical restraints, and medications. Here are some of the study findings.

➤ Alzheimer's disease is more than twice as common in SCU residents.
➤ Surprisingly, SCU residents have less stroke and congestive heart failure.
➤ Physical disability is less common in SCU residents.
➤ SCU residents have more mental disabilities,

indicated by hallucinations and the use of psychotropic drugs.

The researchers found that it costs less to care for residents in an SCU than other residents in the same facility. But they also found that facilities without an SCU had lower staffing costs than facilities with them. "We speculate that the SCU-containing facilities in our sample, chosen in concert with the Alzheimer's Association, may be more oriented toward providing a high-quality service," they explain. "Regardless of actual costs, some evidence exists that charges are higher for SCUs." Mehr and his colleagues conclude that more research is needed on Special Care Units and the outcomes of this care.

The Fine Print

Caregivers need to read the fine print on medical insurance forms. You may be surprised by what's covered and what isn't. Mom's insurer will pay for root canal work but not dental extractions. Other insurers may pay for only a portion of ambulance charges. Not only do family caregivers have to take up the financial slack, but they also have to submit reams of paperwork.

At one point, Mom was transported to the local hospital by ambulance. The bill arrived the following week. Immediate payment was required, and the company would submit the paperwork to the insurance company. Several weeks later I received a letter denying payment. It seems that the person at the ambulance company who copied Mom's insurance number had copied it incorrectly. Although I was reimbursed, the experience was unsettling.

My husband and I haven't figured out how much we spend on Mom, and we never will. She doesn't need much, but socks get lost, slippers get misplaced, and underwear gets ragged. We pay for these and other items, such as postage and Christmas gifts. It's the least we can do for Mom at this time of her life.

Some family caregivers invest substantial sums in home remodeling. Special ramps may have to be built for wheelchair patients, for example. The patient may need a walker or a hospital bed. If the family caregiver works outside the home, he or she may have to hire a sitter to stay with the patient. The patient may spend part of the day at an adult day care center, which can run from twenty-five to one hundred dollars per week.

All of these costs add up. Tracking care costs is time-consuming and confusing. Caregivers need to be aware of the patient's basic costs and the extra costs. These costs should be spelled out in assisted living and nursing home agreements. Don't sign any agreement until you understand the costs involved.

Basic Fees

Jo Horne, the author of *The Nursing Home Handbook: A Guide for Families,* says the basic nursing home fee should cover the patient's room, meals/snacks, housekeeping, linen (but not personal laundry), nursing care, custodial care, and keeping medical records. The fee should also include paperwork necessary for hospital transfer. Payment falls under Title XIX guidelines, Horne points out, and "currently pays for 41.8 percent of the care given older persons in nursing homes."

Because of nursing home reforms passed in 1987, Horne says, they "cannot require you as a family member to sign a contract agreeing to guarantee or pay as a third party for care for a defined period of time before the resident starts to receive Title XIX."

Extras

Some nursing homes are segmenting their services to compensate for the rising costs of care. Extras may include the services of ophthalmologists, dentists, podiatrists, physical therapists, speech therapists, and laboratory workers. Beauty and barber shop fees may be extra. In some nursing homes, help with feeding is an extra cost. The patient's special diet may also be considered an extra.

Saving Costs with Volunteer Services

Thanks to dedicated volunteers, many hospitals, assisted living communities, and nursing homes are able to offer more extras to their residents at no cost. Volunteers give manicures to females residents in Mom's nursing home. Mom loves to get a manicure because she can't do it herself, and it's one-to-one contact. Other volunteers come in to play music and read stories. If you can't volunteer your own time, you may help by donating magazines or funds.

Using volunteers is a way to contain costs, but there are advantages for the volunteers, too. They learn more about the facility and the residents who live there, and they derive satisfaction from helping others. If you would like to volunteer your time and talents, contact the facility directly, or check your newspaper for a list of facilities with volunteer programs.

SOURCES OF REVENUE

There are five basic sources of revenue to pay for patient care. Katherine L. Karr discusses these sources in her book *Promises to Keep: The Family's Role in Nursing Home Care.* Personal finances are one source. However, a family with limited income, property, savings, and investments may only be able to afford a few months of care. Karr suggests that you choose a licensed home that accepts Medicaid patients so you won't have to move the patient again when your funds run out.

Private health insurance is the next means of payment. Karr asks family members to examine each policy's benefits before purchase. Does the policy meet all of the patient's needs?

Nursing home care may also be covered under veterans' benefits. In other words, the patient is housed in a nursing home that has a contract with the Veterans' Administration. Then there's Medicare. "Medicare payments are strictly limited to persons placed in nursing homes for specific, treatable conditions," explains Karr. She says only a small percentage of existing nursing homes qualify for these payments. Skilled nursing services, such as insulin injections, are covered, but custodial services, such as bathing, are not. Medicare will pay for up to one hundred days of care, depending on a physician's diagnosis.

More About Medicare

Medicare payments cover daily skilled care only. As Seth B. Goldsmith points out in his book *Choosing a Nursing Home,* Medicare has specific requirements:

➤ The services must be ordered by a physician.

➤ The services must be provided by health professionals (nurses, physical therapists, speech pathologists).

➤ The services must be needed on a daily basis.

➤ The services must be provided in response to a condition that required hospitalization.

The 1996 Guide to Health Insurance for People with Medicare, published by the U.S. Department of Health and Human Services, spells out Medicare clearly. Who qualifies? People who are at least sixty-five years old, people (of any age) with permanent kidney failure, and other disabled people under age sixty-five. Medicare Part A is financed by Social Security funds and the Self-Employment Tax. Medicare Part B is partially financed by premiums paid by enrolled participants.

Lisa Berger discusses Medicare payments in her book *Feathering Your Nest: The Retirement Planner.* "Medicare is a bare-bones policy," she explains. What are the differences between Part A and Part B? Berger says Part A pertains to *hospital* insurance and that anyone over age sixty-five who is eligible for Social Security gets it.

Part B pertains to *medical* insurance: doctors' fees, outpatient services. Funds come from the U.S. Treasury and the beneficiary's monthly premium, and services must be provided by a medical doctor or a doctor of osteopathy. Only one chiropractic service is covered by Medicare—manipulating the spine to correct a dislocation revealed on an X-ray. Medicare doesn't pay for X-rays that are taken by a chiropractor.

Your Medicare Handbook by the U.S. Department of Health and Human Services explains, "Medicare Part B picks up where Part A leaves off." Payment depends on many criteria, including benefit periods, reserve days, and the type of facility. Here's the basic payment plan.

PART A:	PART B:
➤ Hospitalization	➤ Medical expenses
➤ Skilled nursing care	➤ Clinical laboratory services
➤ Home health care	➤ Home health care
➤ Hospice care	➤ Outpatient hospital treatment
➤ Blood transfusions	➤ Blood transfusions
	➤ Ambulatory surgical services

Physician's services are covered wherever the patient receives them, whether in a nursing home or a hospital. Part B helps to pay for a variety of related services, such as physical or occupational therapy, flu shots, mammograms, oxygen equipment, wheelchairs, and walkers.

If Medicare denies payment to the patient for services,

family caregivers have the right to appeal on behalf of the patient. There are specific steps to the appeal process. Contact the Medicare carrier or intermediary in your state for more information. *Your Medicare Handbook* contains a state-by-state list of Medicare carriers and their toll-free phone numbers. You can also look in your phone book under "U.S. Government" for the office nearest you.

Medigap

You may want to buy additional insurance to fill in the gaps in the patient's coverage. This Medigap insurance is regulated by federal and state laws. The National Association of Insurance Commissioners developed ten standard Medigap plans, which were given letter names to signify their different benefits. Plan A is basic insurance, and Plan J is the most comprehensive.

All of the states offer Plan A insurance. However, some states prohibit certain plans, and others limit the number that are available. Minnesota, Massachusetts, and Wisconsin have different Medigap plans because they passed legislation before the federal standards were in place. Under federal law, states are allowed to add on benefits. Contact your state office for more information.

Medicaid

Don't confuse Medicaid with Medicare. Medicaid is a federal reimbursement plan for people with low incomes. In order to qualify for Medicaid, the patient may not have more than two to three thousand dollars in assets (state laws vary). Application forms are available at county government offices. The form is long and detailed.

Extensive documentation is needed, so apply early, when the patient has about eight thousand dollars. A county financial advisor can help you to fill out the form.

Before the patient is eligible for Medicaid, the caregiving spouse must spend down their joint assets. Burial fees may be paid ahead of time. In case Mom died while I was out of town, I signed a document called "My Personal Funeral Arrangements Made with _____ Funeral Home." I also signed an Irrevocable Burial Form. This form names the funeral home as trustee and sets aside up to two thousand dollars for funeral expenses.

The funeral home supplied both documents. Keep in mind, however, that the Irrevocable Burial Form doesn't include transportation costs. If the patient's body has to be shipped to another state, burial costs will be higher. Family members will have to set aside these funds beforehand. The funds must cover the basic service charge, pick up and delivery, opening and closing the grave, a vault for the casket, and the grave marker.

LEGAL DOCUMENTS

Because of the way forms are processed, the health care provider may overpay family caregivers. This has happened to me several times with the Mayo Clinic and funds have been returned to me. In order to receive a refund you may be asked to supply a photocopy of your power of attorney form. I keep a supply of photocopies on hand for this purpose.

Family caregivers should also have other documents on hand, including:
➤ The patient's will;
➤ Any loan documents;
➤ Income tax returns;
➤ Pay receipts;
➤ Social Security documents;
➤ Credit card statements;
➤ Life insurance plans/certificates;
➤ Medical insurance information;
➤ Retirement benefits (medical and dental);
➤ A list of assets;

➤ Any safe deposit box number;
➤ Appraisals.

Having these documents will help you manage the patient's finances and, more important, prove your management. Look around the patient's residence carefully before you move him or her into a nursing home. When I cleaned out Mom's studio apartment, I found a receipt for a cemetery plot under her bed. I worried about the documents I didn't find.

FUTURE COSTS OF CARE

In a recent issue of the *University of Minnesota Medical Bulletin*, Peggy Rinard reported that four million older Americans suffer from Alzheimer's disease. The cost of their care is a hundred billion dollars each year. Most of these costs are for nursing home and long-term care. All too often, the patient's funds are depleted by the time he or she reaches the later stages of the disease.

Although some states report more cases than others, the total number of Alzheimer's cases in the country is rising. People with any chronic illness have lots of bills. According to a recent article, "Chronic Conditions a Huge Burden on Health Spending," which was published in the *American Medical News*, the number of patients with chronic illness is rising. By the year 2030, care costs will shoot up to $798 billion, and those costs were figured in 1991 dollars.

Who knows what the care costs will be in the years ahead? Catherine Hoffman, ScD, and her colleagues examine costs in their paper "Persons With Chronic Conditions: Their Prevalence and Costs."

"The chances of becoming a caregiver are greater now than ever with long life expectancy, the growing numbers of persons over the age of 85 years, and the limited network of potential caregivers because of small family sizes," they say. Unfortunately, as the researchers note, our health care systems are largely based on acute illness, not chronic illness. Alzheimer's is a chronic illness that—as our society is quickly realizing—affects nearly every family in America. There are financial programs to help families pay for the cost of Alzheimer's care. Minnesota is a progressive state, willing to help the disadvantaged and the needy. However, some families have taken advantage of this by hiding the patient's assets, moving him or her to another state, and applying for financial aid. This is fraud.

FRAUD

You can help cut down on fraud by checking Medicare bills for errors, calling about questions, and being suspicious. As *Your Medicare Handbook* points out, be suspicious if you're offered free testing, screening, or medical equipment in exchange for your Social Security number, or if someone representing the government tries to sell you something.

One entry in Mom's check register was for a fourteen-dollar check to a Social Security protection agency. Was this a scam? I called the local Social Security office. The representative who answered knew exactly what I was talking about. "Oh, gosh," he said. "I haven't heard about these for a few years."

"It sounds like a scam to me," I interrupted.

"I know it does, but it isn't illegal," he replied. "The companies are asking for contributions. It's voluntary."

"But the people are going to get their Social Security money anyway," I countered.

"Yes, but the companies say they will make sure the trust funds will be saved for you for the rest of your life," he explained. "Some companies promise to lobby a senator or congressman."

Admittedly, Mom's check was a small contribution. If thousands of confused people sent in that much, however, the company was doing well.

We need to protect Alzheimer's patients from schemes, scams, and fraud. Assisted living facilities and nursing homes may have to hire bonded financial advisors to do this. Financial reimbursement plans were set up to help the needy, not the greedy. Let's use these systems fairly. When fraud is committed, all of us wind up paying.

What Can You Do?

Read medical policies carefully.

Get financial counseling.

Determine the patient's basic care costs.

Become aware of extra costs and track them.

Budget for these extra costs, if possible.

Keep good financial records.

Become a nursing home volunteer.

Know the difference between Medicare and Medicaid.

Know the difference between Medicare Plan A and Plan B.

Project the patient's future care costs as best as you can.

Help stop fraud.

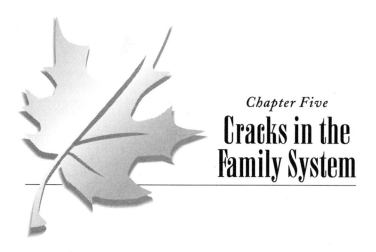

Chapter Five

Cracks in the Family System

Alzheimer's disease changes the patient's personality. These changes may be gradual or sudden. I realized that dementia had erased the two dominant traits of my mother's personality—intelligence and humor. The pain of this discovery is beyond words.

Mom's intelligence and humor have been the mainstays of my life and I counted on them. Thinking about her sense of humor brings back a childhood memory. For years Mom had wanted an apple tree. Dad finally bought her a small sapling, and she planted it in the center of the yard, away from the rear garden.

The tree was so skinny it looked like a rake handle in the dirt. But Mom had high hopes for the tree and its future harvest. That night, under the cover of darkness, she snuck into the backyard and tied bright red apples onto the tree branches. She discovered the "miracle" in the morning and told our neighbors about it.

The neighbors laughed heartily when they saw the tree. I chuckled every time I looked out the kitchen window. This story evokes poignant feelings because that heroine, someone I knew and loved and admired, has become a stranger. Still, as hard as it has been, I've had time to adjust to these changes.

Adjustment doesn't mean the absence of pain. I've struggled with Mom's changed personality, her odd mannerisms, and her behavior disturbances, each one a crack in the family system. These cracks may be divided into two groups: patient and caregiver. Let's start with the patient, who comes first.

CHANGES IN THE PATIENT

Personality

Changes in the patient's personality are more shocking if they happen quickly. Researcher U. M. Mann and his colleagues write about rapidly progressing Alzheimer's in a letter to *The Lancet*. They summarize their recent research at the National Institutes of Health in Bethesda, Maryland. Forty-six patients with probable Alzheimer's disease were given various mental tests. Mann and his colleagues concluded that Alzheimer's patients may fall into two groups: slow clinical progression, and fast progression of dementia.

My mother's progression has been slow. All of the family caregivers that I've talked with said they were disturbed by the changes in their loved one's personality. Despite all of my caregiving efforts, I'm always out of step with Mom. Just when I think I've caught up with her, she changes again.

Anjan Chatterjee, MD, and his colleagues, authors of "Personality Changes in Alzheimer's Disease," think personality changes in patients aren't well understood. They studied thirty-eight patients from the Alzheimer's Disease Registry at the University Hospitals of Cleveland, Ohio. A caregiver completed a personality inventory on each patient twice—once to describe the patient before probable Alzheimer's disease, and once to describe the patient after onset.

The inventory focused on five aspects of personality: neuroticism, extroversion, openness, agreeableness, and conscientiousness. According to the researchers, "The largest changes were decreases in reported conscientiousness and extroversion, along with an increase in neuroticism."

The caregivers thought Alzheimer's made the patients more anxious, depressed, and vulnerable. As you might expect, patients with paranoid delusions were considered more hostile.

The researchers say Alzheimer's patients may converge into an "AD [Alzheimer's Disease] personality, with a reduction in the normal variability of personality traits." Reduction is a kind word, I think, not representative of the changes I witnessed. There have actually been times when I've been afraid of my own mother.

Changes in Mannerisms

Changes in mannerisms often parallel changes in personality. If you've ever visited a nursing home you're aware of these mannerisms. Some patients are constantly calling out. Others keep clearing their throats. Still others are rocking back and forth. Then there's foot tapping and tapping on surfaces with fingers.

Mannerisms can be annoying to watch. My mother developed so many mannerisms I could hardly keep track of them. Before dinner was ready, Mom would sit down at the table. Evidently, the waiting taxed her patience, and she would tap her feet. If I had put anything on the table, such as applesauce, she would start eating.

She would also keep wiping her eyebrow with her finger. I'd never seen her do this before. This mannerism became a part of her conversation. But the worst mannerism of all was her purring. Mom would purr as regularly as a coffee pot. The final mannerism was head-bobbing, an indication of neurological damage.

Observing these mannerisms was painful because they symbolized a failing mind. What fails first? According to doctors, the general rule is that the highest centers of the brain go first—names, phone numbers, facts. However, recent brain research is making some doctors question this theory.

Behavior Disturbances

I remember Mom as a beautiful woman, inside and outside, who treated others with kindness. Anger was rare and when she got angry, it was for a good reason. Now her anger was like smoldering ashes, ready to ignite at any minute. Mom even staged tantrums to get her own way.

The agreeable mother of my past became a master of manipulation. She was also good at laying on guilt. "Whenever I call, you're not home." "You said we'd go shopping." "I haven't had a new dress in years." (Untrue, but Mom believed it.) From my perspective, it looked like all of Mom's remaining intelligence was being put to poor use.

D. P. Devanand, MD, and his colleagues discuss behavior changes in their paper "Behavioral Syndromes in Alzheimer's Disease." They describe their work with the Behavior Syndromes Scale for Dementia (BSSD), which examines five behavior changes.

1. Disinhibition (wandering, going into other resident's rooms, and impulsive behavior, such as Mom buying the new Cougar).
2. Catastrophic reactions (crying jags, profound anxiety, and anger).
3. Apathy/indifference (few facial expressions, speaking in a monotone voice, a disinterest in activities).
4. Sundowning (late-afternoon or early evening agitation).
5. Denial ("There's nothing wrong with me!").

Two thirds of the patients they studied denied having any memory problems. Reading this finding made me think of Mom. Several times she told me, "Thank God I don't have that mental disease, you know, the one where you forget. Ants-hammer's or Antsheimer's. I'm not sure what it's called."

Aggression. Dr. Devanand and his colleagues found that approximately one-fifth of the patients were aggressive. Verbal aggression was more common than physical aggression. Mom exhibited both types and got into several fistfights with another resident of the nursing home who, as she said, "drives me nuts." Several times she threw things across the room.

Her verbal aggression increased rapidly. I took her out to lunch every Wednesday. At first, we went to various restaurants, but this upset Mom, so I chose one restaurant. As Mom became more demented, she became more concerned about entrances and exits. "How the hell do you get out of here?" she'd ask.

In response, I asked the hostess to seat us near the door. Mom would then watch the people in line and make nasty comments. "Look at how fat she is!" "That's some getup he's wearing." "Is that a foreigner?" Some of her comments made me want to hide under the table.

At least her physical and verbal aggression were signs of spirit. Then one day her personality sputtered and went out like a flickering light bulb. Mom rarely smiled anymore, and her voice was devoid of inflection. The few sentences she said were short, comprised of nouns and verbs, with an occasional adjective.

Physical aggression can tax a caregiver's skill. One winter day I decided to visit Mom. Just as I was about to enter the nursing home, two caregivers wheeled an elderly man outside. He was screaming at the top of his lungs and trying to hit them.

Since I'd talked with the resident several times, I approached his wheelchair. "Hello," I said.

"Watch out!" a caregiver cautioned. "He might hit you."

Sure enough, the man's hand nearly connected with my face. I see now that I shouldn't have interfered. After a few minutes in the cold, fresh air, the man calmed down. When

I left the nursing home he was asleep in his wheelchair. This goes without saying but I'll say it anyway: a caregiver should never hit a patient.

Apathy. Apathetic patients are less interested in activities and personal care. They also look and sound apathetic. Looking back, I realize Mom's apathy started more than nine years ago. I had called to tell her our older daughter had been involved in a near-fatal car crash. "That's too bad," Mom said in a casual voice.

"She has a broken neck, a blood clot on the brain, and wedged vertebrae," I continued, trying not to cry.

"Oh," Mom said, and changed the subject to shopping. I was devastated. Tragedy had struck our family, and I wanted my mother's comfort. Instead, I got total disinterest. At that moment, I realized Mom was incapable of understanding the severity of any situation. I never sought her comfort again.

CHANGES IN THE CAREGIVER

Role Reversal

Finally, Mom developed what doctors call a "flat affect," or absence of personality. Although I didn't want it to happen, I found myself reversing roles with her. This didn't change our biological relationship. Mom will always be my parent and I will always be her daughter. Although reversing roles with her was necessary, it was as painful as wearing ill-fitting shoes. Neither of us were comfortable with the arrangement.

Reversing roles made Mom angry, and she would scream, "You're not my mother! I can do what I want." Despite getting lost countless times and developing a tendency to fall, she refused to wear an identification bracelet. "Why should I wear that?" Mom asked. "I know my own name."

Family caregivers described their roles on the CNN television special "Alzheimer's: The Long Good-bye." A patient's wife said, "I feel most of the time I'm in a cage and the bars are coming closer."

A daughter said, "Changing his diapers is not good for me."

Another wife said, "I think I'm coming to the end of my rope...there's only so much I can do."

To get another slant on role reversal, not just my own, I called a friend of mine. "We actually dole out money to my mother a few dollars at a time," she said. It seems her mother carried money in a small purse and was losing ten- and twenty-dollar bills. "I remember when my mother doled out money to me," my friend said thoughtfully.

Toileting problems caused another form of role reversal for my friend. "My mother has bladder urgency," she explained, "so I started buying pads for her." Instead of throwing the pads away, her mother was reusing them, sometimes washing them, and hiding them. "I tried to find the pads, but I know I missed some," she said.

Laundry created another form of role reversal. The daughter did her mother's laundry each week and put the clean clothes away. "I'm going to be really honest here," the daughter said. "I ask myself, 'How many more weeks or years am I going to be doing her laundry?'" Reversing roles with a parent is painful and tiring.

Loneliness

Sometimes, one adult child in the family is selected as the family caregiver and the others may not get involved at all. This puts a greater burden on the caregiver. It may also isolate the caregiver from family members. Research findings show loneliness is also a problem for many spousal caregivers. As many have discovered, loneliness can exact a high psychological toll on caregivers.

Loneliness is detailed in the paper "Alzheimer's and Related Disorders: Loneliness, Depression, and Social Support of Spousal Caregivers." Author Brenda Bergman-Evans, RNC, PhD, thinks caregiver loneliness is a serious mental health problem. Moreover, she thinks our society adds to the problem. "In America, being married, having friends, and other indications of sociability are signs of success; being isolated and friendless are signs of failure," she notes.

Spousal caregivers lose more than companionship. Forced isolation may also cause them to lose touch with their friends. There are only so many hours in a day, and many family caregivers are confined to their homes. Bergman-Evans points out that some research shows that younger spousal caregivers are even lonelier than older ones. Because loneliness is a subjective feeling, she urges readers to view these findings cautiously.

There's more to the loneliness issue. Edna L. Ballard, MSW, ACSW, and Cornelia M. Poer, BA, explore this issue in their book *Sexuality and the Alzheimer's Patient.* Friends and family members may shun the caregiver because they don't want to "buy into" his or her psychological pain. "People pull away because they are embarrassed or afraid of the changes they see in an old friend," the authors explain.

What can you do about loneliness? Each caregiver has to find his or her own ways of coping. Here are some practical suggestions:

1. Set up a buddy system and stay in touch with your buddy. My dearest friend and I, who were both caring for failing parents, became a mutual support system. She always understood what I was saying and had encouraging words for me. I was happy to support her, as well.

2. Contact the Alzheimer's Association and sign up for

their newsletter. Also, ask for their book list. The Minnesota Alzheimer's Association has an ongoing list of recommended reading. They sell these resources at conferences, or you can order them by phone.

3. Join a support group. You may not be able to attend every group meeting, but at least you know you have some support. The friends you make could turn out to be your friends for life.

4. Do something for yourself. Every caregiver needs some time off. Reward yourself by going out to lunch, seeing the latest movie, or window shopping. Getting away can renew your soul.

Being the Only Caregiver

Often the Alzheimer's patient has only one caregiver. Being the only caregiver is hard. The title of an article in the newsletter *Day by Day: Caring For Patients With Alzheimer's* offers good advice: "Always Keep a Helping Hand Within Easy Reach."

The article advises caregivers to take some time off every once in a while. Leave the Alzheimer's patient with a trusted relative, friend, or day care program. What's more, caregivers need to take care of themselves. How you do this is a personal choice.

Being the only caregiver can cause not just a crack but a fissure in the family system. "I get so tired," one caregiver explained. "My brother lives only an hour away. He never calls my mother. He never writes to her. He's glad I'm doing all of the work."

Alzheimer's disease is the kind of health crisis that enhances or damages family dynamics. Herbert N. Budnick, PhD, focuses on family dynamics in his book *Heart to Heart: A Guide to the Psychological Aspects of Heart Disease*. Although he writes about heart disease, his insights also apply here.

Budnick tells how he drew a diagram of his family.

According to Budnick, drawing a family diagram can help you learn more about your family. Start by drawing a circle to represent the family unit. Add family members to the inside of the circle, depending on how you interact with and relate to them. Then draw lines between various family members to indicate their relationship. Use one line to show a weak bond and two lines to show a strong bond.

When Budnick drew his own family diagram, he showed a weak bond between his father and himself—one line. Helping people, doctors, nurses, technicians, and hospitals were listed outside the circle.

When I drew the family diagram, the strongest bond was between my husband and me. Instead of being on the outside of the circle, Mom's doctor and the director of nursing at the nursing home were on the inside, almost like family. Your family role—leader, follower, clown, super-responsible member—may also influence your diagram.

The Executive Personality

Alzheimer's is usually a disease of the elderly, and adult children are caring for their parents at a time when their own careers are peaking. Health professionals are becoming more aware of executives who are caregivers and their need to "straighten everyone out."

One executive became furious at his father's doctor. "I've taken three days off to come here," he exclaimed. "This is taking too much time." The executive threatened to report the doctor to his superiors. What the executive failed to realize is that medical tests, especially tests for Alzheimer's disease, take time.

Executives may also be long-distance caregivers. Trying to rush the medical tests doesn't help the patient. In fact, the patient may pick up on the executive caregiver's stress. To make matters worse, the executive may be used to giving orders and may start ordering health professionals around. But the tactics that work in industry may not work in medicine.

The executive may also be feeling guilty for not doing more for the patient. Job responsibilities may divert the caregiver's attention. Often the executive is pulled in opposite directions—stretched to the limit and ready to snap. Add money worries to this picture and you understand the magnitude of the problem.

Being an Alzheimer's caregiver is a career in itself. This means that the executive caregiver has dual careers. While some manage to strike a balance between the two, it's a constant juggling act. Something has to give, and often that's self-care. See chapter 10 for more information on this topic.

Fatigue

Family caregivers often complain of fatigue. "If I'm this tired now, what will I be like in a year?" asked one caregiver. Holidays can be especially stressful for caregivers. Even the caregivers who know how to pace themselves may not be able to do so.

Many of the caregivers I've talked with complain of sleep problems. Their worries wake them up in the middle of the night. One worry leads to another, and hours later the caregiver is still awake. Authors Nancy L. Mace and Peter V. Rabins, MD, point out in their book *The 36-Hour Day*, that fatigue can be a sign of depression.

Sleep-deprived caregivers are easily exhausted. The caregiver is constantly trying to adjust his or her life to the patient's life—a balancing act that doesn't balance. It will never balance. Anne Boykin, PhD, RN, and Jill Winland-Brown, EdD, RN, presented their study in an article called "The Dark Side of Caring: Challenges of Caregiving."

For this study, five family caregivers were asked to respond to this statement: "Please describe your experience of being a caregiver for your relative with Alzheimer's disease. Share all thoughts, perceptions, and feelings until you have no more to say about the experience." The caregivers received no prompting other than the query, "Can you say more about that?"

The interviews were done privately, recorded, and transcribed. Four themes emerged from the interview data.

1. Frustration and self-sacrifice.
2. The need to share caregiving experiences.
3. The stress of dealing with the patient's altered reality (including the inability to understand time).
4. The caregiver's guilt.

One of the husbands talked about his fatigue and said his wife had developed a pattern of going to bed, getting up to dress, undressing again, and repeating this pattern throughout the night. Another husband expressed concern about his wife's nighttime wandering—a worry that hardly promotes sleep. It's easy to understand why some researchers think Alzheimer's disease has *two* major victims, the patient and the caregiver.

Anger

Tired and stressed caregivers tend to be angry caregivers. You may be angry at people who don't do things on time or who fail to follow through. You may be angry at other family members who aren't "tied down" with caregiving. You may be angry at the disease itself. And as Jo Horne writes in *Caregiving: Helping an Aging Loved One,* "You may also become angry with yourself for your imagined failings as a caregiver."

Horne says caregivers must understand that anger is a normal response. I believe this. Yet, anger is a stressful emotion. Once, when Mom called me to say she had bought clothes at the mall, I felt myself flush with anger. "You don't need any more clothes," I screamed. "Stop spending money!"

The next morning my husband and I went over to Mom's townhouse and we had a terrible confrontation. My explanations and logic had no effect on Mom, so I took her checkbook away. I also removed charge cards from her wallet. What did Mom do? She opened a new charge account at a major department store.

Talk about anger! I went to the store and closed the new account. "Why are you giving charge accounts to demented old ladies?" I asked. "I closed this account once, and I'm closing it again. What's more, I will not pay for any purchases charged to the account."

I also called our lawyer. He said I might have to contact the major stores and ask them not to sell anything to Mom. Thank goodness I didn't have to do this. Closing one account seemed to put a damper on Mom's spending—that action, and my watchful eyes.

Jo Horne doesn't think caregivers should always hide their anger. "You are both human, and that person needs to see that sometimes you have needs also," she writes. I guess my anger needed to come out. Life doesn't always give us the choices. My only choice was to conserve Mom's funds, but I still feel guilty about our confrontation.

Guilt

Guilt can cause major cracks in the family system. The son who is constantly traveling and rarely visits his mother may feel guilty for his lifestyle. The daughter who is the primary family caregiver may feel guilty about the anger she feels. Hard as she tries, this anger doesn't go away. Members of the extended family may struggle with feelings of guilt, too.

In "The Dark Side of Caring: Challenges of Caregiving," Boykin and Winland-Brown say it's hard to handle guilt and respect the patient's dignity. "Most caregivers experienced feelings of guilt for treating their loved one as a child or for responding angrily in vulnerable moments," they write.

All of us have our vulnerable moments. Talking about the weather would start an argument when Mom was feeling combative. Although I fought against it, I found myself getting angry at her. Immediately, I would feel guilty for reacting this way.

Fortunately, I was able to get past these feelings. I took no pride in this progress, however. Getting past my anger had more to do with Mom's failing IQ than my own character. Still, it made my caregiving easier. What are the sources of guilt, and how do they affect us?

Guilt Sources. According to Hanns G. Pieper, PhD, author of *The Nursing Home Primer: A Comprehensive Guide to Nursing Homes and Other Long-Term Care Options,* guilt has several complex sources. First, we may have some stereotypes about nursing homes. Rather than thinking of the nursing home as a secure, comfortable place, we may see it as a sign of personal failure. We failed to take good care of someone we love.

In the past, so-called "maiden aunts" used to take care of family members. Today there are few maiden aunts, and they're probably at work. When they're at work, they may feel guilty for not being at home with the patient. When they're home, they may feel guilty for wanting to be at work, away from the caregiving routine.

The patient's feelings can also make a caregiver feel guilty. As Pieper explains, "Your mother, if she is opposed to the nursing home, may add to your guilt by reminding you that she took care of you and that her friend Emmy Lou is living in her daughter's house, and furthermore, if you really loved her, you wouldn't put her away in a nursing home."

Pieper explains that other family members may also add to the caregiver's guilt. Siblings who aren't helping out may feel guilty about their lack of involvement. As Pieper says, "They're feeling guilty too, and one way they have of handling the guilt is to dump it on you since you have assumed the tremendous responsibility for your mother's care." The key words here are *tremendous responsibility.*

In fact, the growing responsibilities of caregiving may cause the family to fracture. The family may break into two separate parts: me (the main caregiver) and you (other family members). Once this mindset has been established, it's hard to stop it. Family disagreements may continue long after the patient's death.

Marital Relationships

Spousal caregivers find themselves in a new and strange relationship. How did the familiar become unfamiliar?

One of the most painful results of Alzheimer's is loss of personality. First, the spousal caregiver feels a loss of partnership. In years gone by, the husband and wife were a couple. Suddenly, with Alzheimer's, what used to be two is now one. The word "we" may no longer describe your life. A second person may live in the house, but the caregiver is essentially flying solo. It's very difficult for spousal caregivers to deal with this kind of pain.

There's also a loss of companionship. Perhaps the couple belonged to a weekly bridge club. Over time, the patient not only forgets how to play bridge, he or she doesn't know what to do with playing cards. Conversing with the patient also gets harder and harder.

David Eskes discusses marriage in his article "Holding Back the Sunset." He tells the story of sixty-two-year old Don Bliss and his wife, Roxy. At first doctors thought Roxy had a brain tumor. However, other clues led to a diagnosis of probable Alzheimer's.

Because he felt they were a team, Don tried to accommodate his wife's needs. Yet the team grew farther apart. To help his wife find her car, Don bought her an amethyst-colored Cadillac. If they were traveling, he timed their bathroom stops. Because Roxy felt better when she was well-dressed, he bought her more coordinating outfits. He dressed and bathed her and talked with her about their four children.

"The hardest part for a caregiver is the quiet," Don said. "It kills you."

Alzheimer's disease also affects sexual relationships. The patient may have a diminished interest in sex or an excessive interest in sex. Despite advancing disease, Alzheimer's patients may still be compatible with their mates. The next chapter, "I Have a Boyfriend," contains more information on this topic.

Luke Shockman writes about one couple's love and determination in his article "Alzheimer's: Losing Time." "Like most people with Alzheimer's disease, time is slowly being stolen from Dorothy Erickson," writes Shockman. But Shockman thinks the Erickson's story isn't a story of despair; it's a story of determination.

Berdine Erickson accommodated his wife's needs. To help her make choices, he removed many of the clothes from her closet. He drew a line on the bathtub to help Dorothy step into the empty space. Hardest of all, Berdine remembers to smile at his wife when he talks to her. Along the way, he's taken care of himself by attending programs at the Mayo Clinic's Alzheimer's Disease Center. Twice a month he attends a men's support group. He reads about Alzheimer's disease and has many books on the subject. In addition, he started keeping a journal.

The article includes two of Berdine's journal entries, and they're enough to make you cry. One entry tells how Berdine feels blessed. The other talks about his challenges as a spousal caregiver. "I must try as a caregiver to help her live her life in a sense by walking in her shoes and doing what she can't do by herself." Berdine says that this is an awesome responsibility.

DIVIDING GOODS

Many caregivers find their responsibilities awesome and divisive. That's why a friend suggested I write an entire book about dividing up the goods. I didn't do it, but her point is well taken. Dividing up the goods is more about feelings than possessions.

However, the task is inevitable. The time comes when the family members have to meet, dismantle the patient's household, and decide what to do with the belongings. Families have been torn apart in the process. Dividing Mom's goods wasn't a problem for me because my brother and I agreed on things beforehand. Other families haven't been as fortunate.

Edward Myers discusses family strife in his book *When Parents Die*. "The problem is rarely a matter of greed," he observes. "It's usually more [a matter of] the belongings' sentimental value." Myers points out that siblings may fight over the same item. One sibling may want to keep items in the family, whereas others may want to sell them. "To argue over the dollar value of belongings is beside the point," summarizes Myers.

Dividing the goods is harder if you don't have an inventory of the patient's things. Insurance companies can give you leads on how to do this efficiently. Look in your local bookstore for other resources. You might want to divide up the inventory tasks to make the process easier. The important thing is to have a written inventory and a plan.

Don't follow the examples of my mother and my aunts, who devised a note system. They stuck notes on items or beneath them, indicating who was to receive the item. Unfortunately, notes have a way of coming off and getting lost. What's more, the people who find the notes may not follow them.

My aunt died alone in her Florida condominium. Other residents of the high-rise realized they hadn't seen her in a day and called the police. When the police entered her condominium, they found my aunt on the floor. She had posted notes around the apartment, and one said the diamond ring on her hand was to go to me. According to other residents, the police had been in the apartment for three hours.

The ring was never found, and other valuables were missing. A relative went to Florida to investigate and filed a complaint with the police department—to no avail. I don't care about the diamond ring, but I'm furious and sick at heart at what the loss represents. What kind of people rob the dead?

Besides creating an inventory of possessions, the family members need to agree on some sort of plan. One family used a number allocation plan to disburse goods. Valuable items, such as antiques and furniture, were given numbers. A drawing was held to see who would get these items. This plan worked for them and may also work for you.

As we've seen, cracks in the family system may be patient-based or caregiver-based. Despite these cracks, the family may continue to function. It may not function efficiently, but the family structure can remain in place. With time and patience, cracks in the family system may be repaired with love, the glue that holds families together. You can also hold yourself together by taking these action steps.

What Can You Do?

Prepare for changes in the patient's personality.

Prepare for behavior disturbances and find ways to handle them.

Despite the patient's apathy, live each caregiving day to the fullest.

Set up a buddy system to counter loneliness.

Join an Alzheimer's support group.

Get away for a while.

Let yourself get angry at times.

Identify some sources of guilt.

Keep a journal to identify and track your thoughts.

Inventory the patient's possessions and make a family plan for disbursing them.

Repair cracks in the family system with love and caring.

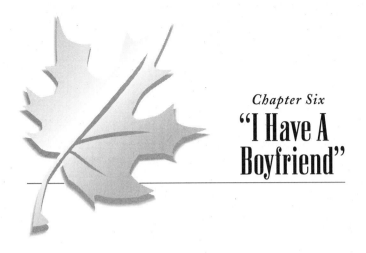

Chapter Six

"I Have A Boyfriend"

I was exiting the highway when Mom announced, "You know, I have a boyfriend."

Her statement was such a shock I almost drove into a light pole. Ideas raced through my mind. Had someone been bothering Mom? Had she been bothering someone? Was she lonelier than I thought? For once in my life, I was speechless.

"He always says hello to me," Mom continued, "and tells me I look nice."

As I pulled to a stop in front of the retirement community, Mom exclaimed, "There he is!"

She was pointing at a priest. I had met him before, and he was a smiling, friendly, and gregarious person. He was also a kind man, and I didn't doubt that he had complimented Mom. It's too bad that she viewed his friendliness in a different way. On the other hand, Mom may have meant that she had a new friend who happened to be male.

For years our society has pretended that older people aren't sexual. They don't have sexual thoughts or sexual feelings, and certainly they don't have intercourse. Yet sexuality is part of being alive; it's nature's assurance that life will continue. Not much attention was paid to the effects of dementia on sexuality until recently.

SEXUALITY IN OLDER PEOPLE

The American culture seems to be obsessed with sexuality. Sex sells products. However, older people are rarely portrayed as sexual beings in these ads. When they are, it's often in a demeaning way that borders on ridicule. Look at some of the recent television commercials and you'll see what I mean.

Nancy L. Mace and Peter V. Rabins, MD, authors of *The 36-Hour Day*, point out that "While our culture seems to be saturated with talk about sex, it is the sexuality of the beautiful and the young that is being discussed." Few people want to think about sexuality in older people, let alone discuss it.

Sexuality in Alzheimer's patients is an uncomfortable, misunderstood, and controversial topic.

All caregivers—professional, family, spousal, and community—must deal with sexuality sooner or later. Where do we start? Mary Petrie, RN, of the Alzheimer's Unit at University Good Samaritan Health Care Center in Minneapolis, thinks we start with attitude. Speaking at an Alzheimer's conference in Winona, Minnesota, Petrie said she was against the term "inappropriate sexual behavior." She also said only 5 to 7 percent of the residents in nursing homes exhibit sexual behavior. This matches the research done by Fernando G. Bozzola, MD, and his colleagues.

In their paper "Personality Changes In Alzheimer's Disease," Bozzola and his colleagues say "sexual misdemeanor" was the least frequent personality change. Of the eighty patients the researchers studied, only 3.8 percent had "sexual misdemeanor." Nevertheless, caregivers need to be prepared for this behavior in case it happens.

SEXUAL BEHAVIOR
AS AN EXPRESSION OF SELF

Sexual behavior in Alzheimer's patients is an expression of self at a time when that self is disappearing. Understanding this behavior is easier if you think of it as an affirmation of life. What is the patient telling us? "I'm alive. I have feelings. I have sexual feelings."

When you think about it, sexuality starts with the mind. A medical essay published by the Mayo Clinic, "Sexuality and Aging," describes the brain as a sexual organ. Sexual stimulation usually starts with the external stimulation of the senses—touch, sight, smell, and hearing. Sexuality is alive and well in the aging population, according to the essay. "The reality is that many older people enjoy an active sex life that is often better than their sex life in early adulthood," notes the essay.

Helen D. Davies, MS, RNCS, and her colleagues discuss sexual issues in their article "Til Death Do Us Part: Intimacy and Sexuality in the Marriages of Alzheimer's Patients." Sexuality concerns are a frequent topic of discussion in Alzheimer's support groups, the researchers say, and concerns range from distress about sexual overtures to fear of inappropriate social behavior such as masturbation. "Despite these concerns, many couples would like to maintain intimate sexual contact," the authors write.

The Patient's Losses

Edna L. Ballard and Cornelia M. Poer, coauthors of *Sexuality and the Alzheimer's Patient,* think the patient's profound losses also contribute to sexual behavior. "The person with Alzheimer's disease, despite his level of impairment, is particularly sensitive to his losses," they explain. It's natural for the patient to compensate for these losses.

There are many practical reasons for sexual behavior. These include:

➤ Needing to go to the bathroom;
➤ Tight-fitting clothing;
➤ A lack of tactile stimulation;
➤ Being too hot or too cold;
➤ Skin dryness or a rash;
➤ Disorientation (patient is confused about time, place, and clothing).

Furthermore, patients may remember getting dressed at one time or another and may not know they're in the dining room and not in their bedroom. Familiar things, such as the chest of drawers Mom brought with her to nursing care, may convince the patient that he or she is at home and not in a public place, where it's not appropriate to walk to the bathroom nude.

Heavy blankets may be another cause of sexual behavior. Patients throw off heavy, scratchy blankets. While sexual behavior challenges all caregivers, it may challenge spousal caregivers the most. Being a spousal caregiver is one of the hardest jobs in the world.

SPOUSAL CAREGIVERS AND SEXUALITY

Although divorce is more common today, it was less common several decades ago. Research findings show that spousal caregivers honor their marriage vows, especially the words "in sickness and in health." Spousal caregivers look to their vows as a source of strength. But, it can be tough going for spousal caregivers, especially for those who have little or no support.

Helen D. Davies and her colleagues write about spousal caregiving in their article, "Til Death Do Us Part: Intimacy and Sexuality in the Marriages of Alzheimer's Patients." They say, "When AD [Alzheimer's disease] strikes, a spouse with these commitments is faced with a situation that, in terms of sexuality at least, is fraught with problematic contradictions." Not only are there contradictions, but spousal caregivers must also grapple with some pretty tough questions:

> ➤ How will it feel to have sex with someone who doesn't know my name?
> ➤ Does my spouse have any inkling of what he or she is doing?
> ➤ Can my spouse or I handle sexual arousal that has no completion?
> ➤ Are there other satisfactory ways to express my love?
> ➤ Does my partner remember intercourse?
> ➤ Will my spouse's sexual talk and behavior hurt any children?
> ➤ How can I divert public sexual behavior?

There aren't any easy answers to questions such as these. Furthermore, the spousal caregiver can't predict his or her partner's sexual behavior. Berdine Erickson wrote about his wife, Dorothy, in the journal entry quoted previously. The entry states that Berdine's wife hopes her disease won't get to the point where she doesn't know her husband.

That hasn't happened yet, but when it does, Berdine is ready. "I have a tremendous loyalty to my wife," he said. Berdine isn't alone. Most spousal caregivers have tremendous loyalty to their partners and, in some instances, their former partners.

One divorced caregiver took her ex-husband back into her home. "He's very confused and has nowhere else to go," she explained. "Sometimes he thinks he's still my husband and sometimes he doesn't. It doesn't make much difference. I'm there and that calms him."

Sexuality in Alzheimer's patients is a complex issue. For many spousal caregivers, this is a bittersweet time. While they want to be with the person they love, that person is slipping away physically and mentally. How do you take care of a dying person and manage to smile?

Vacant eyes and incontinence can be sexual turnoffs. Some spousal caregivers admit to losing interest in their partners. Others say they can't meet the patient's increasing sexual demands and continue to meet the demands of caregiving. And some females admit to submitting to their husbands because they feel it's their duty.

Carol Wolfe Konek writes about attending an Alzheimer's support group in her memoir, *Daddyboy*. During the support group meeting, a spousal caregiver said her husband stopped making love in the middle of intercourse because he had forgotten what he was doing and he had forgotten his wife. The caregiver said she felt "like a prostitute."

Helen D. Davies and her colleagues studied the sexual response patterns in couples and the factors that led to their responses. They discovered that Alzheimer's disease and aging affects male erections. It's more difficult for a male patient to have an erection and sustain it. Although they don't know why this happens, the researchers think the part of the brain that controls erections may be damaged. Sexual therapy has helped some patients, according to the researchers.

SEXUAL BEHAVIOR IN NURSING HOMES

The professional caregivers who work in nursing homes see all sorts of sexual behavior in patients. Yet research shows that many professional caregivers try to avoid the topic of sexuality altogether. Their excuses have some merit:

➤ "That's not part of my job."
➤ "I'm not a sex therapist."
➤ "I'm afraid of him."

In truth, sexuality in Alzheimer's patients can't be avoided. Alzheimer's patients have sexual feelings, behaviors, and memories. Yet sexual behavior can challenge the professional caregivers who work in nursing homes, starting with the fact that nursing homes are public places.

Nursing homes have male and female residents. They also have mixed cases—patients with debilitating illnesses mixed in with Alzheimer's patients. As Mary Petrie explained at the Winona Alzheimer's conference, a male patient may climb into bed with a female patient because she looks like his deceased wife, "the person he slept with for fifty years." And from the patient's perspective, this is a normal response.

Maybe the patient is looking for physical closeness. It's comforting to snuggle up to another person when you're confused and scared.

Maybe the patient is cold and doesn't know how to push the call button to ask for another blanket. The patient may also be looking for good, old-fashioned friendship.

As more and more of the patient's friends die, this need becomes more acute. The authors of *The 36-Hour Day* explain, "Confused persons may become close friends with another resident, often without a sexual relationship. Friendship is a universal need that does not stop when one becomes demented."

On the other hand, masturbating in public, making sexual comments to the staff, and public nudity are all problem behaviors. Combine these behaviors with wandering and you've got real problems. After Mom started to wander, I asked an administrator to explain the retirement community's policies to me. The administrator said they would tolerate some in-house wandering, and some inappropriate language, but not public nudity. Although Mom wasn't very modest, at least she wasn't walking around in her "birthday suit."

TOUCH: A BASIC NEED

I had expected her to stop talking about a boyfriend once she went to nursing care, but she didn't. It seems Mom had found another boyfriend, someone who, she said, "touched my hand." What was going on?

Someone may have touched her hand accidentally or reached out to her in a gesture of friendship. All I know is that the boyfriend idea continued until she lost the ability to create meaningful sentences. Talking about a boyfriend seemed to comfort Mom. I was interested in her need for a boyfriend, someone of the opposite sex who appreciated her.

Despite being in her nineties, Mom was still an attractive woman, a woman who enjoyed having her hair done and wearing flashy clothes. "Don't buy me any more tailored clothes," she kept saying. "You wear that stuff but I don't. I like blouses with ruffles, you know, more dressy clothes."

Many of the clothes in her closet were made of swishy fabrics: silk, silk look-alikes, and rayon. Although I wouldn't wear most of her clothes, I could understand how Mom would like them. Touch is a powerful sensation, and her clothing selections may have been influenced by the way the fabric felt on her skin.

Humans have an instinctive need to be touched. In fact, babies who are deprived of touch quickly develop psychological problems. Touch deprivation can have harmful effects on Alzheimer's patients, too. Helen Davies and her colleagues write about touch in their paper "Til Death Do Us Part: Intimacy and Sexuality in the Marriages of Alzheimer's Patients."

They say touch "elicits a sense of generalized relaxation that makes caring and sharing natural." How can we give patients the touching they crave? The book *Sexuality and the Alzheimer's Patient* contains a list of ways, and I have added to it. Touch experiences include:

➤ Taking the patient's pulse;
➤ Holding and patting hands;
➤ Putting on hand lotion or powder;
➤ Cutting, combing, and washing the patient's hair;

➤ Bathing the patient (if he or she isn't afraid of water);

➤ Shaving the patient;

➤ Dancing or tapping feet with the patient;

➤ Engaging the patient in a range of motion exercises;

➤ Playing tactile games, such as balloon ball (catching a large ball while sitting in a circle);

➤ Using pet therapy;

➤ Treating the patient with certain occupational/physical therapies.

The authors say, "Care must be taken to be aware and respect those individuals who do not want (and may never have liked) to be touched except by a small circle of intimates." Caregivers must also remember to touch frail and severely ill patients gently.

Reading about the need for touch reminded me of the time I styled Mom's hair. During one of her infamous Minnesota visits, the wind destroyed her hairstyle. I offered to restyle it with a curling iron. She didn't seem to know what a curling iron was, but I could tell she enjoyed having her hair touched.

"See, I'll put a few curls on this side," I said. "Now I'll put some curls on the other side."

She kept turning her head to see the results of my efforts. After I'd finished styling her hair, I unplugged the curling iron and started to walk away. Mom didn't move. She stood in front of the mirror in a trance. I don't think she wanted the physical contact to end. Turning away from the mirror she said, "I look old on the outside, but I feel young on the inside."

Dressing patients is another way of touching them. Even when Mom could still button clothing, she kept asking me to do it for her. "You didn't button my coat all the way up," she would say. She also liked me to pull up the hood and tie a scarf beneath her chin. Of course, I hugged her afterwards.

PROBLEM BEHAVIORS

Despite touch activities, the Alzheimer's patient may still exhibit problem behavior. Let's consider these behaviors and what can be done about them. According to the authors of *Sexuality and the Alzheimer's Patient* problem behaviors include:

➤ Fondling breasts in public;

➤ Public nudity;

➤ Exposed genitals (the patient's fly may be unzipped);

➤ Masturbation;

➤ Inappropriate sexual comments;

➤ Pressing genitals in public;

➤ Urinating or defecating in public.

To this list I would add exposing breasts. The patient's breasts may be exposed because her blouse wasn't buttoned correctly or the buttons came undone. Mom has worn gaping blouses and put her slacks on backwards, with the zipper wide open. She was totally unaware of these things.

Patients may also share sexual thoughts with a caregiver, which can be inappropriate. At least, this was problem behavior for me. One spring I drove to Iowa to pick up our daughter at college. Much to my surprise, Mom decided to come along. I was even more surprised when she started to share her sexual memories with me. Since I didn't want to hear about my parents' sexual exploits, I kept quiet, hoping she'd stop if I didn't encourage her. This hint went unnoticed and she continued her story, ending with the words, "I got pregnant."

Still I said nothing. What could I say? Mom interpreted my silence as approval and continued with her story. Despite my embarrassment, I learned something that I'd never known; she had suffered two miscarriages. I think Mom was remembering all of her children, the unborn, born, and the twin who died.

"He was so little, under three pounds," she said wistfully. "Too little to live. I couldn't go to the cemetery to bury him. Your father took care of all of that." Mom was thinking about the stream of life—her marriage, sexuality, parenthood, and a death she could never forget.

Helping the Patient

There are no all-purpose rules when it comes to sexuality in Alzheimer's patients. Each patient must be considered on an individual basis. Talk with the patient's doctor about sexuality. You might want to fill out the questionnaire on page 54 of *Sexuality and the Alzheimer's Patient,* a book by Edna L. Ballard, MSW, ACSW, and Cornelia Poer, BA, if you're a spousal caregiver.

The yes-or-no questions cover sexual issues and patient health. A sample question: "Incontinence is a problem for me/my spouse; it affects my feelings about sexual relations." Questions like this are useful because they help the spousal caregiver take stock of things. With the doctor's help, a plan can be worked out that helps both patient and caregiver.

Be Informed

All caregivers need to be informed about sexuality in Alzheimer's patients. The Minnesota Alzheimer's Association rents videos about sexuality, and I watched *A Thousand Tomorrows: Intimacy, Sexuality and Alzheimer's,* produced by Terra Nova Films in Chicago. In the video, spousal caregivers talk candidly about sexuality issues.

What impressed me most about the caregivers was their love for their spouses. Their love was so abundant, so touching, I found myself rummaging in my purse for tissues. The video showed the richness of their love—the kind of love that lasts right up to the end, and beyond death.

Computer databases such as *Medline* are another source

of information. An article in the *American Medical News*, "What's the Deal With All This Free Medline?" compiled by Nina Sandlin describes *Medline* as the "largest single-subject database" in the world. A service of the National Library of Medicine, the *Medline* database contains more than eight million references. As impressive as this is, there seem to be few resources on sexuality in Alzheimer's patients. More research is needed, particularly on the effects of medication. The information may be difficult to obtain; anecdotal research needs to be done carefully because the patient may have fragmented or false memories. The research needs to be interpreted carefully as well.

Respect Privacy

Experts recommend private rooms for couples in nursing homes. If one spouse lives in a nursing home and the other does not, private settings should be provided for these couples to visit together. Private settings give couples a chance to hug and kiss and talk. The couple may sit in a lounge or walk in the garden when others aren't around.

We can also respect the patient's privacy by closing the door, drawing bed curtains, using folding screens, and providing private dressing areas. These steps ensure privacy and show that we respect the patient's dignity.

Touch Experiences

Experts say that touch should be part of the patient's care plan. You might want to give the patient daily back rubs or massages. Before you start, make sure the patient doesn't have any bed sores. Also, check with a doctor if the patient is recovering from surgery. Follow the touch suggestions listed previously.

I noticed that Mom became less aware of touch experiences as she became more demented. She would fall asleep while she was having her hair shampooed. Because she didn't recognize the family members, sometimes she would pull away if we came too close. Mom needed to be touched, but it was getting harder to touch her.

Some days the patient may withdraw, like Mom, and other days the patient may permit touching. Caregivers need to be adaptive and intuitive, and should continue to provide the patient with touch experiences. Some patients have benefited from holding and caring for a doll.

Involve Family

Mary Petrie, RN, of the Alzheimer's Unit, University Good Samaritan Health Care Center in Minneapolis, involves family members in sexuality issues and planning. First, a social worker talks with family members about their sexuality comfort level. Then a Sexuality Intervention Plan is drawn up according to the family's guidelines. For example, family members may not wish to be contacted if their loved one hugs another nursing home resident. The plan starts with the question, "Should we intervene?"

An administrator activates the plan if the answer to this question is "Yes." Suppose a nude female patient left her room, found a walker, and walked the full length of the nursing home hallway. I have filled in the Sexuality Intervention Plan with a real-life example from a nursing care home.

Sexuality Intervention Plan
Intervene?
Yes

➤ Stop/Prevent further activity

Put robe on patient and assign care plan staff person to watch her.

➤ Document incident

Nude patient pushed walker down hallway. Visitors saw her.

➤ Notify family

Called daughter on 2-28-97.

➤ Communicate to Care Plan Team

Make sure patient is dressed when she leaves her room. Give walker to patient after she is dressed. Put noise monitor on. (A noise monitor helps professional caregivers track the patient's moves. Not all nursing homes have them.)

"We try to create a psychologically safe environment," Petrie says. She adds, "A caregiver should never scold a patient." Scolding doesn't help the situation and may do the patient more harm than good. Rather, caregivers should provide the patient with an affectionate and understanding environment. The caregiver also needs to remain calm.

Petrie suggests using same-sex caregivers and dressing the patient in clothing that is harder for the patient to take off. The caregiver may buckle the patient's belt in the back, for example, or put suspenders on slacks.

The authors of *Sexuality and the Alzheimer's Patient* think timing the patient's baths may help to curtail sexual behavior. "Caregivers may find that giving warm baths to the patient before bed is more arousing to the patient than giving a bath in the morning or afternoon," note the authors. Family caregivers should check with nursing home administrators to see when baths are given and request a change if necessary.

Family caregivers may also turn to professionals for help with sexuality issues. In addition to contacting the patient's family physician, you may contact a psychiatrist, psychiatric nurse, psychologist, social worker, sex therapist, and support groups. Talk to other family caregivers, too, because they are fountains of practical information.

Tips for Caregivers

What can you do if things get out of hand? Here are five tips from personal experience:

1. Assess the situation. Is this a sexuality problem or something else? Step out of the picture mentally to see what's really going on.

2. Leave for a few minutes. Ask someone else to supervise the patient, leave for a few minutes, and return. When you return, the patient may have calmed down and may already be thinking about something else.

3. Divert the patient. Try to get the patient involved in an activity, such as looking at magazines or listening to music on a headset. Diversion works, but you have to time it right and have the right diversion.

4. Praise and encourage acceptable behaviors. Tell the patient that he or she is kind, helpful, friendly, and so on. If you're not a family caregiver, ask permission to give the patient a hug. Praise acceptable behavior and try to ignore the less acceptable.

5. Contact professionals. To learn more about sexuality, contact the Alzheimer's Association; the American Geriatric Society; the American Association of Sex Educators, Counselors and Therapists; or the Sex Information and Education Council of the U.S.

Despite a lack of medical proof, I'm convinced that sexuality in Alzheimer's patients and those with other forms of dementia is one of the last things to go. Mom would bring up sexual topics when she could still verbalize her thoughts. One day she asked suddenly, "I wonder how they did it?"

"Who are you talking about, Mom?" I asked.

"Our neighbors. I wonder how they did it."

"Did what?"

"You know—had sex. I wonder how they did it. I can't

picture _____ and _____ having sex."

"Well, they probably couldn't picture you having sex either," I replied. Mom chuckled.

After my father died, Mom seemed to have a yearning in her soul, a need that couldn't be satisfied. She expressed this need in an unusual way. Every time she visited us, Mom brought a small jewelry case. The case was crammed. "Your father gave me this," she would say, lifting a pin out of the case, "and he gave me this."

One by one, she took each piece out of the case and laid it on the table. The jewelry show became a ritual. It evoked pleasant memories and proved that someone had loved her. Mom's favorite piece was a gold charm bracelet with her grandchildren's names on it.

On Christmas morning in 1996, my husband and I and our younger daughter went to visit Mom. With our few presents in hand (new socks and a practical cardigan sweatshirt), we approached her reclining chair. Although she didn't know us, seeing my husband brought a rare sparkle to her eyes. "You're a guy," she declared.

This was the first sentence I'd heard her say in weeks. Mom mumbled something about "looking good," and then her speech failed. We didn't know what was going through her mind. Mom seemed to be lost in the past. Maybe she recognized my husband or was remembering the special guy—the only guy—in her life.

What Can You Do?

Consider sexuality as an affirmation of life.

Look for practical causes of sexual behavior, such as tight-fitting clothes.

Include touch in the patient's care plan.

Identify the patients who don't like to be touched.

Find ways to deal with problem behaviors.

With the family's help, make a Sexuality Intervention Plan.

Talk with the patient's doctor about sexuality.

Assess and reassess the situation.

Divert the patient's attention.

Praise some behaviors and ignore others.

Contact sexual associations and groups.

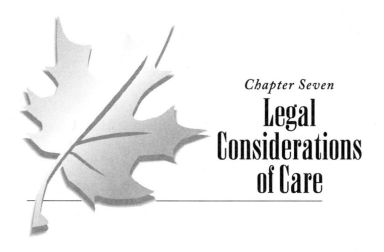

Chapter Seven

Legal Considerations of Care

In addition to monitoring the patient's medical status, the family caregiver must monitor his or her legal status. Start early because you can't predict how quickly the disease will progress. "Prompt action will also let you know the person's wishes are being respected and will relieve you of the burden of second-guessing [legal matters] later the disease process," writes Marilynn Larkin in her book *When Someone You Love Has Alzheimer's*.

This is excellent advice. Unfortunately, Mom's independent nature prevented me from following it. Because I was a long-distance caregiver I didn't know she had been bilked out of thousands of dollars. Mom never told me about her financial losses. With the loss of these dollars came the loss of her dreams.

LOST DOLLARS, LOST DREAMS

Years ago Mom invested fifteen thousand dollars in the Government National Mortgage Association, commonly called Ginnie Maes, a sound investment. In her book, *Feathering Your Nest: The Retirement Planner*, Lisa Berger explains that Ginnie Maes are fixed-rate home mortgages, pooled together and insured by the government. "If an individual homeowner defaults, the government, not Ginnie Mae investors, swallows the loss," writes Berger.

It turned out that Mom had not invested in Ginnie Maes. The company was actually a Ponzi scheme and investors' funds were used to buy rundown real estate. Occasional dividends were mailed to placate investors. Mom received three small checks, one followed by a letter saying the dividend had been paid to her by mistake. My kind, honest, church-going mother mailed it back.

Three hundred investors, all bilked out of their investment funds, filed a class-action lawsuit. Mom was already involved in the lawsuit when I took over the management of her finances.

I had little documentation, however—only a lawyer's assurance of Mom's fifteen thousand dollar investment. Then something strange and amazing happened. While I was writing this chapter, I decided to look through Mom's files for heading ideas. The files had been chaotic when I first received them and had been moved five times.

You can imagine my surprise when I saw a folder caught beneath the others. There were lots of papers in the folder—receipts, photocopies of canceled checks, and carbon copies of personal correspondence. Yet I couldn't piece the story together. Using Post-It notes, I put a date on every piece of paper in the file, and arranged the documents in a time line on the kitchen counter.

Like a photographic negative developing, a plot unfolded before my eyes, with a story line as gripping as any mystery novel. And it had the elements of a good mystery—malice, greed, and fraud. Mom hadn't lost fifteen thousand dollars; she had lost fifty thousand dollars!

How had she gotten involved? In 1984, Mom received a letter from a brokerage house citing the advantages of investing in government-backed mortgages. The letter said the mortgages were safe, had a high yield, offered a monthly dividend check, and had liquidity. Photocopies of newspaper articles about government-backed mortgages had been sent with the letter.

I found three checks made out to the brokerage house.

Other documents showed that eventually the FBI had become involved. Mom had tried to get her money back, joining the class-action law suit and writing to her senator, her congressman, and her broker.

The letters were written on an old typewriter and carbon copied on onion skin paper.

Reading the letters brought tears to my eyes. One letter to the broker says, "To date I have not received the certificate....I would appreciate hearing from you on this matter." Mom signed the letter, "Cordially." Another letter to a law firm reads:

> *Gentlemen:*
> *Enclosed copies are self explanatory.*
> *I am an 81 year old woman and depend on this income for my livelihood.*
> *I was under the false impression that this registration statement was government insured.*
> *Would appreciate your advice on this matter.*

The file wasn't just evidence of a failed investment, it was evidence of a failing mind. As the dates progress, Mom's handwriting gets shakier. Scribbled notes are crossed out.

I realized that Mom remembered one check and forgot the other two. Eventually the state of Florida charged the company with fraud, and a court trustee was appointed to investigate the case.

The trustee's document describes the properties that were purchased with investors' money. A rental property was over-encumbered with debt, a construction project had legally entangled loans, a motel investment might get entangled in litigation, and some funds had been used to buy a plane. For years the case has been tied up in the courts.

Mom received two small compensation checks. A third was due, and the case was coming to a close. With days to spare, I called the Florida Comptroller's Office and faxed eighteen pages of documents to prove Mom's investment. I wanted to stand up for both of my parents, who had worked hard for every dollar they earned. The claims coordinator who was handling the case responded quickly by phone, fax, and letter. Since no previous claim had been made on two of Mom's investments, no compensation could be awarded under the current case. However, the claims coordinator set up a new claim based on the information I had sent her.

Mom may be gone by the time this claim is settled. I wished she had never moved away from Long Island. I ' wished I had been there to monitor her investments. I wished I had been a better caregiver. Still, I was glad I had followed our lawyer's advice and gotten Mom's power of attorney.

POWERS OF ATTORNEY

Conventional Power of Attorney

There are several kinds of powers of attorney. Each is obtained under different circumstances and each has distinct advantages. A conventional power of attorney gives another person the temporary right to manage someone else's financial affairs.

Dennis Clifford, the author of *The Power of Attorney Book* says the conventional power of attorney may be restricted to a major transaction such as selling a car and expires on the date cited on the document. He says a conventional power of attorney is "a useful legal method to authorize the handling of many short-term financial and business matters when the principal [person creating the document] won't be available." The person who gets the power of attorney is called the attorney-in-fact.

Durable Power of Attorney

Because Alzheimer's is a progressive disease, experts think family caregivers should get a durable power of attorney. This document gives a relative or concerned person the legal right to make financial and medical decisions if the patient is incapacitated. Durable power of attorney is valid when the patient is disabled or mentally incapacitated. According to Clifford, a durable power of attorney "normally terminates only if the principal dies or revokes it."

"Legal Considerations for Alzheimer's Patients," a brochure published by the Alzheimer's Association, notes that the patient "must, at the time of drafting and signing the document, have cognitive ability and an understanding of the responsibilities and powers being conveyed." I have a short-form power of attorney for my mother. The document grants me power to act in Mom's behalf. It covers:

➤ Property transactions;
➤ Personal property transactions;
➤ Bond, share, and commodity transactions;
➤ Banking;
➤ Business transactions;
➤ Insurance;
➤ Beneficiary transactions;
➤ Gifts;
➤ Fiduciary transactions;
➤ Claims and litigation;
➤ Family maintenance;
➤ Military service benefits;
➤ Written documents.

I thought Mom might not sign the power of attorney document. Our lawyer said he was used to working with elderly and confused people and told me not to worry. He began the meeting by saying he had gotten his mother's power of attorney. Mom thought our attorney was so charming she tried to sell him her car.

"Do you want to buy my Cougar?" she asked. "It's black and has big tires and leather seats."

I was embarrassed by Mom's hard-sell tactics, but our lawyer was amused. Most important, when we left the lawyer's office, Mom seemed to be pleased. "I'm going to look out for you," I said. "Anybody that tries to cheat you or get your money will have to go through me." Of course, I didn't yet know she already had been swindled out of fifty thousand dollars .

"Springing" Durable Power of Attorney

There's another type of document that family caregivers may want to get, a "springing" durable power of attorney. It's a safety valve for the future. If the person becomes incapacitated, then, and only then, does the document take effect. If the person doesn't become incapacitated, the document is void. Alzheimer's caregivers rarely obtain this legal document. Here's a summary chart about powers of attorney.

Power of Attorney (POA)

Conventional POA Grants another person the right to manage the patient's affairs.

Durable POA Grants another person the right to manage the patient's legal and financial affairs before and after the patient is incapacitated.

"Springing" Durable POA Grants another person future rights to manage the patient's financial and legal affairs when and if the person becomes incapacitated.

I ordered new checks with Mom's name and my name printed on them, and the letters POA beside my name. Getting Mom's power of attorney went smoothly for me. Other family caregivers aren't as fortunate. A mentally incompetent patient may refuse to sign the power of attorney document. In this case, the family caregiver may have to get legal guardianship, which is also called legal conservatorship. Let's take a brief look at the guardianship process and how it works.

GUARDIANSHIP

A court hearing is held to determine if the patient is capable of managing his or her own affairs. If the patient is found to be incapacitated, a judge assigns a guardian to that person. Be aware that patients in the early stage of Alzheimer's may be able to convince a judge of their competency. The patient may rally for the occasion and gain the judge's sympathy.

Marilynn Larkin writes about guardianships in her book, *When Someone You Love Has Alzheimer's*. She points out that the conservator must file periodic reports to the court about the patient's finances. She adds, "If there is a dispute among family members about the individual's care, some states require a guardianship of the person to give a court order that the care be provided."

HEALTH CARE PROXY

A health care proxy provides another way for caregivers to help the patient. This legal document authorizes a spouse, adult child, or other concerned person to make health care decisions for the Alzheimer's patient. A health care proxy covers all medical decisions, not just those that involve life-support systems.

Caregivers should keep in mind, however, that a health care proxy doesn't cover any financial decisions. As author Marilynn Larkin notes in her book *When Someone You Love Has Alzheimer's*, having a proxy can prevent expensive court proceedings and delays in medical treatment.

ADVANCE DIRECTIVES

For all caregivers, advance directives are a crucial part of patient care. The directives cover a wide range of treatment issues. Joanne Heathman, RN, CS, GNP, of Mayo's Department of Community Internal Medicine, spells out these directives in the program notes for the Third Annual Mayo Alzheimer's Disease Center Conference for Families.

Heathman says there are two types of advance directives. First, there's the treatment directive. This directive includes the patient's living will and a "do not resuscitate" order. Second, there's the patient's proxy directive, which is actually a power of attorney. Advance directives also:

➤ Allow the patient to decide who should make medical decisions;

➤ Take effect when the patient is incapable of making decisions;

➤ Apply only if the patient is mentally incapacitated;

➤ Help others to make decisions for the patient;

➤ Can be changed or canceled;

➤ May be verbal as well as written;

➤ May be reviewed by an attorney;

➤ Must be witnessed.

State law requires nursing home administrators in Minnesota to check the patient's advance directives on a regular basis. At every care conference I'm asked if the "do not resuscitate" order is valid. My answer is always "Yes." Hard as it is to discuss these things, I know I must do it for Mom's sake.

"Do Not Resuscitate" Order

Not long ago Mom fell against a wall, hit the floor, and broke her nose. An ambulance took her to the trauma center at a local hospital. Following correct medical procedure, Mom's physician asked if I had a "do not resuscitate" order.

"Yes," I said. "That's what my mother wants."

I was asked about the order again when Mom was transferred to her hospital room. A doctor or nurse would ask me about the order every time I visited her.

This was mental torture for me because I had to make the same painful decision over and over again.

When I answered "Yes" to the inquiries I was really in turmoil. My intellectual self was answering the question affirmatively, but my emotional self was answering the question negatively. I wanted the doctors and nurses to revive my mother. I wanted her to see the millennium, to experience life in the next century, to live forever.

Yet I was legally and morally bound to yield to Mom's request for no unnecessary measures. I kept telling myself that Mom had lived a long and interesting life. These mental assurances didn't erase the pain I felt. In fact, the emotional pain of caregiving got worse.

PATIENT LIABILITY

Are family members legally responsible if the patient injures someone else? That was the question recently asked in a Wisconsin courtroom. The case was detailed in an article called "Patient with Alzheimer's Not Responsible for Injuring Nurse."

An elderly male patient was convicted of injuring a female nurse. She had found the patient in the wrong room and, as she directed him to the right room, the patient struck her. The nurse sued the family. Despite the fact that the patient had been diagnosed with probable Alzheimer's and was living in a Special Care Unit, the jury was asked to disregard this information.

This was the crux of the case. The court's directive "prevented the jury from establishing whether the patient had control over his behavior," the article explains. Obviously, an Alzheimer's patient has no control over his or her behavior, and the case was overturned.

I wondered about liability after Mom said she was going to volunteer to work in a hospital gift shop. She was living in the retirement community at the time, and a staff member had suggested the idea because Mom was so bored. Although I tried to stall Mom, she became fixated on the idea and talked about it often.

"I'll probably start next week," she said.

I called the staff member. "Volunteering in the hospital gift shop is a good idea," I said, "but it isn't a good idea for my mother. She can't read numbers, can't make change, and can't track inventory. What can we do?"

The staff member said she would call Mom in a few days and tell her the volunteer positions were filled. Mom was disappointed by the news. Within a few weeks, though, she had forgotten about the gift shop and was off on another tangent. I was very relieved.

LEGAL ADVICE

State laws vary, and the patient may be liable for things in one state and absolved in another. Many family caregivers can't pay for legal advice, but, you may get free legal assistance from the Legal Aid, a federally funded program.

The person applying for legal assistance must bring supporting documents to prove need. These documents include income tax returns (federal and state), Social Security verification, and any other forms of government assistance you may be receiving.

Contact the National Alzheimer's Association for more information on legal advice and options. Ask for the brochure "Legal Considerations for Alzheimer's Patients."

Your state association may have special materials as well. For example, the Minnesota Alzheimer's Association has put together a medical assistance kit that contains a summary of eligibility rules.

You may also get legal advice from:

➤ Legal Services for the Elderly
130 West 42nd St., 17th Floor
New York, NY 10036

➤ National Senior Citizens Law Center
1424 16th Street NW, Suite 300
Washington, DC 20036

➤ AARP Legal Counsel for the Elderly
1090 K Street NW
Washington, DC 20049

➤ American Bar Association
750 North Lake Shore Drive
Chicago, IL, 60611

Before you write or call, check a recent phone directory and the toll-free directory for the most up-to-date addresses and phone numbers. Take notes during phone conversations. Date and file all of the legal advice you receive.

LEGAL DOCUMENTS

Family caregivers should gather the patient's legal documents together and store them in a safe place. Your local Alzheimer's Association can help you do this. To prevent loss, I glued small receipts and papers to letter-size paper with Post-It glue. All documents should be labeled clearly.

I am constantly amazed at the number of documents, receipts, letters, and forms that I have for Mom. When she was living in Florida, Mom sent me the location of her safe deposit box, its number, and a duplicate key. Now I have her documents in our safe deposit box. What documents should you have?

➤ A birth certificate (an original or a duplicate).
➤ A will.
➤ Any life insurance policies.
➤ A cemetery plot certificate.

➤ Trust document(s).

➤ A power of attorney document.

➤ The names, addresses, and phone numbers of relatives and friends to notify at time of death.

➤ Income tax records.

➤ Canceled checks.

Photocopy all documents, including the patient's death certificate when the time comes. Experts recommend getting at least twelve copies of the death certificate. Family caregivers will need these to process the patient's will and for other legal considerations.

Gathering documents is a painful and time-consuming process. Jo Horne writes in her book *Caregiving: Helping an Aging Loved One*, "The key is to make sure that these financial and legal matters are handled as early in the caregiving process as possible."

Just because you've gathered these documents together doesn't mean your work is done. The family caregiver may have to submit more documents to various agencies. For example, Mom's Social Security check is deposited directly into her bank account. As her power of attorney, I am required to fill out forms on how the Social Security funds are spent.

I'm glad the Social Security Administration is protecting my mother. Ken Oestreich, of the Social Security Administration, cites some other good ideas in a nationally syndicated article called "Make Sure Your Benefits Will Be There." He asks Social Security recipients to check their W-2 forms to make sure the name and number are correct and keep records up to date.

The Patient's Will

As soon as the patient is diagnosed with probable Alzheimer's, he or she should get a will. Even if the patient has a will, it's a good idea to review it. Mom's will is a simple one, and I have a copy of it in my safe deposit box. Keep in mind that a will must meet certain legal criteria to be valid.

The patient must understand what he or she is allocating—dollars, property, treasured possessions. In addition, the will must tell how these assets are to be distributed.

Moreover, the patient needs to remember who he or she has listed as beneficiaries. And this point may cause some problems.

The patient's lucidity is fleeting. He or she may be lucid on some days and totally forgetful on others. The family caregiver may have to ask a psychiatrist or neurologist to determine the patient's competency. It's better to be safe than sorry.

A Living Trust

A living trust is a financial arrangement. Under this arrangement a person is appointed by the patient to act as his or her trustee and to hold title to assets. However, the trustee must manage these assets according to the terms of the trust document.

How I wish I had a living trust for Mom when she was sucked into the mortgage scam. Maybe I could have prevented these losses. On the other hand, the sellers were so slick I might have been sucked in along with Mom. Anyway, experts think a living trust may help family caregivers avoid costly probate charges.

VALUABLES

Family caregivers may want to remove valuables from the patient's home or room for safekeeping. I hadn't paid much attention to Mom's figurines until my brother commented on their value. He advised me to store them in a different place. This was good advice because it protected the figurines and made Mom's move to nursing care easier.

Mom had a companion who came in twice a week to

straighten up the apartment and help with the laundry. One day the companion called to tell me that Mom had given her a ring "with a large stone in it." Although the ring turned out to be dime-store quality, I removed all of Mom's valuable jewelry from her apartment as well.

SAFE DEPOSIT BOXES

Valuables should be stored in a safe deposit box to protect them from theft, fire, and weather damage. The patient may want his or her own safe deposit box because it's a sign of independence. This decision can cause problems, however. While Mom remembered that she had a safe deposit box, she couldn't remember where it was, and she lost the ability to recognize keys.

What's the solution? The family caregiver may be a joint signer for the safe deposit box. Check with your local bank to make arrangements. If the patient loses his or her key, the bank may have to break into the box at the cosigner's expense.

Keep a list of the documents that are stored in the safe deposit box. Our bank provides its customers with pre-printed forms for this purpose.

The power of attorney document ceases at the time of death. State laws differ, and the patient's power of attorney may be allowed to open the box to remove the patient's will. In some states, a relative is allowed to open the box with a court representative present. A lawyer will be able to answer other questions you may have.

TAXES

When the patient is no longer able to file his or her own taxes, someone must do it for the patient. Often this is the family caregiver who has the patient's power of attorney. Make sure you include a photocopy of the power-of-attorney document with the tax returns. Mom left such a confusing trail of income, investments, and losses that I used a professional tax service.

The manager of the service I chose took a personal interest in my mother. She picked up on deductions that I might not have noticed. Last year, I didn't file because Mom's medical expenses exceeded her income. However, I continue to keep careful financial records for her.

PENDING LEGISLATION

Caregivers shouldn't assume that laws remain the same. Existing legislation may be modified, and new legislation may be introduced that affects the patient. *American Medical News* staff writer Sharon McIlrath details a recent legal controversy in her article "Medigap Under Fire: Can It Be Fixed or Should It Be Ditched?" McIlrath says the issue is a bipartisan one.

Some health care economists think Medigap can be repaired; others want it stopped. Standards for Medigap coverage were established by each state. But McIlrath says the General Accounting Office found "more than a third of all Medigap companies failed to meet these standards in 1993."

Economists are trying to figure out a way to design a fair system that helps the disabled elderly and at the same time, urges them to use Medicare in a prudent way. All caregivers need to stay informed about pending legislation. The legal considerations of caregiving can be confusing, but if we take one issue at a time, we can make sense out of things.

Be kind to yourself and give yourself plenty of time to sort through paperwork. If you get confused, take a short break, and then resume work. Make good use of the legal services available in your community. The time you spend now may save you dollars and cents later.

What Can You Do?

Monitor and review the patient's investments.

Get the patient's power of attorney.

Gather the patient's legal documents together and store them in a safe place.

Photocopy all important documents.

Keep liability issues and events in mind.

Get legal advice when necessary.

Make sure the patient has made out his or her will.

Consider getting a living will to protect the patient financially and legally.

Store the patient's valuables in a safe place.

Store legal documents in a safe deposit box.

Keep up with pending legislation and tax laws.

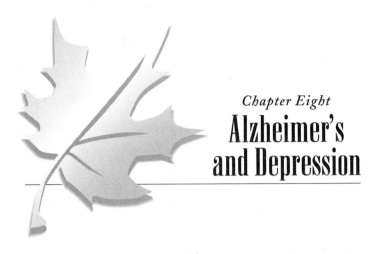

Chapter Eight

Alzheimer's and Depression

Who doesn't have bad days? All of us have times when we feel blue. But feeling blue is different from depression.

The most common type of mental illness in the nation, depression is also the most treatable. Depression can strike anyone, including someone with Alzheimer's disease.

About 25 percent of Alzheimer's patients are depressed, according to Marilynn Larkin, the author of *When Someone You Love Has Alzheimer's*. Depression in the Alzheimer's patient can be difficult to treat. It requires keen medical observation and skill.

WHAT IS DEPRESSION?

The National Alliance for the Mentally Ill defines depression as a type of brain disease. The disease causes the ill person to feel despondent, inadequate, and pessimistic about the future. Depression is "just as much an illness as kidney or heart disease or any other physical disorder you might name," writes Leonard Cammer, MD, in his book *Up From Depression*. Looking at what depression is and isn't will give us a clearer picture of the disease.

Depression isn't the blues. The blues go away and depression doesn't. This isn't to downplay the seriousness of the blues, for these feelings can be harmful. "The blues can be as bad for a life as weeds are for a garden when they obstruct hope, wring out energy, and make us feel terrible," says Malcom Boyd in *Modern Maturity*.

Depression isn't sadness. Over time, sadness gradually decreases, whereas depression gets worse. This puts the patient in danger. Chronic depression can lead to suicidal thoughts and actions. Depression isn't a lack of moral fiber. Many of those afflicted with the disease try valiantly to overcome it. Alzheimer's disease and depression have many symptoms in common. Like Alzheimer's, depression has a noticeable path of progression. The path may be slow or fast.

DISEASE PROGRESSION

Dr. Leonard Cammer describes the progression of the disease in *Up From Depression*. He says depression starts with the blues, but the blues don't go away. Blue feelings turn into black feelings of extreme sadness. Then feelings of helplessness and hopelessness take over the mind.

Aging people are often depressed people, according to the American Association of Retired Persons (AARP). The AARP examines depression in its brochure "Depression Later in Life." The brochure attributes depression in older people to biological and emotional changes.

The brochure also points out that depression isn't typical of aging. However, some older people are overwhelmed by their losses. "When a person is overwhelmed with loss and is unable to cope, depression may become a severe problem," the brochure explains.

Because one disease is superimposed on another, the Alzheimer's caregiver may miss the symptoms of depression.

Experts say depression is part of Alzheimer's—it comes with the territory. Keep the symptoms of Alzheimer's in mind as you read about the symptoms of depression.

SYMPTOMS

The AARP brochure "Depression Later in Life," lists these symptoms of depression, and I have added to them.

➤ Changes in eating and sleeping habits.

➤ Changes in sexuality.
➤ Concentration problems.
➤ Difficulty in making decisions.
➤ Withdrawal from social contacts.
➤ Total disinterest in social contacts.
➤ Preoccupation with aches and pains.
➤ Persistent sadness.
➤ Crying for no apparent reason.
➤ Irritability (and sudden anger).
➤ Decreased energy and listlessness.
➤ Suicidal thoughts and attempts at suicide.

Jo Horne, the author of *Caregiving: Helping an Aging Loved One,* divides the symptoms of depression into three categories: psychological, physical, and verbal. Under the psychological category, she lists reduced pleasure in favorite pastimes, concentration problems, and anxiety. Under the physical category, she lists loss of appetite, tearfulness, and sleep disturbances. Under the verbal category, she lists a quote: "All of my friends are dead."

Seeing that sentence was an eye opener because my mother used almost the same words. "I read the church program to see what's going on," she commented. "I don't know any of the names. All of my friends have died."

I had been aware of Mom's depression for some time and recognized the symptoms. To get a better picture of her depression, I sat down at the kitchen table and listed Mom's symptoms under Horne's categories. Seeing the symptoms on paper gave me a better understanding of her mental state.

Mom's Psychological Symptoms

➤ Irritability/anger.
➤ Stopping favorite activities (bridge, reading).
➤ Boredom.

➤ Apathy.

➤ Hallucinations.

➤ Delusions.

➤ Loss of hope.

Mom's Physical Symptoms

➤ Listlessness.

➤ Constant desire to sleep.

➤ Wandering.

➤ Flat affect (no personality or interest in life events).

➤ Aggression (pushing, hitting).

Mom's Verbal Symptoms

➤ Constant complaining.

➤ "Attack" sentences ("I'm going to biff you!").

➤ Short sentences.

➤ No voice inflections.

➤ Withdrawal from conversation.

Long before she showed signs of dementia, Mom showed signs of depression. I could read it in her letters and hear it in her voice. My father's health was failing and taking care of him wore her out.

A three-pack-per-day smoker, Dad was losing the battle against lung disease. I flew out to Long Island to see him. Dad was frail and Mom wasn't herself; she was disheveled, depressed, and worried. Money was running out and Mom would lose her home if she complied with Medicaid laws. She didn't know what to do.

Dad had been a volunteer fireman and, with the help of other firemen, was admitted to a special nursing home in upstate New York. He died there of the complications of pneumonia.

The Christmas after he died, Mom flew to Rochester. She exited the jetway wearing a black coat, a black hat, a black blouse, black slacks, and black shoes. She was carrying a black purse. "She looks so depressed," I thought to myself. Even when Mom saw me, she didn't smile.

Since then, Mom's depression has gotten worse. I remember her as an honest, outgoing person who shared her thoughts easily. Progressive dementia made it harder and harder for Mom to share her thoughts. As I discovered, some of her thoughts were about suicide.

SUICIDAL THOUGHTS

It was a Wednesday, and I had gone to pick up Mom for lunch. Her apartment window was open, and I could hear robins singing (a sound I loved) and smell freshly mowed grass. Without any warning, lead-in sentence, or words, Mom turned to me and said, "I'm going to jump from that window."

"Don't say that," I answered. "It's a beautiful summer day, and we're going to have a nice lunch together."

"I don't care. I'm going to jump," Mom replied.

Her words frightened me. Although I managed to get Mom out of her black mood, I couldn't get her suicide threat out of my mind. Weeks later, she threatened to commit suicide by taking a bottle of pills. This was as shocking as her threat to jump from the eighth-floor window.

Two days before this second threat, Mom had asked me to buy her a bottle of over-the-counter pain medicine. I had bought the medicine and delivered it to her. If she took all of the pills, Mom could kill herself. Did she have the cognitive ability to plan suicide?

I wasn't sure, but I knew she could do something impulsive. As time progressed, her suicide threats turned into a manipulative tactic. Whenever I refused to give Mom money for something advertised in the newspaper, she would threaten to commit suicide. The threats were frightening and tiring.

Nevertheless, I took Mom's suicide threats seriously and reported them to the retirement community's medical director. I also arranged for her medications to be dispensed by a registered nurse. Gradually, her suicide threats waned.

Suicide threats are more common in the early stages of Alzheimer's. Caregivers need to be alert to the symptoms of suicide. "When Depression Turns Deadly," an article published in *Modern Maturity,* says to watch for extreme sadness, lack of energy, boredom, disinterest in life, desire to sleep, hopeless feelings, anxiety, and talk of suicide.

Why Depression Is Missed

Depression in Alzheimer's patients is so often missed. Why? One reason is that Alzheimer's and depression have many of the same symptoms. Author Katherine L. Karr says depression may masquerade as something else. In her book *Promises To Keep: The Family's Role in Nursing Home Care,* Karr explains that depression can look like agitation—a very different problem from depression.

Family and friends may make the mistake of thinking depression is a natural, unavoidable occurrence in something that happens to older people, according to the AARP. Their brochure "Depression Later in Life" also notes that family and friends may mistake the symptoms of depression for senility.

Older people rarely admit they're depressed, and many try to disguise their feelings. After she moved to Florida, Mom adopted a "fun in the sun" attitude to try to stop her pain. At times her attitude seemed almost frantic. Because she was cut off from everything she knew—family, friends, neighbors, church contacts, community—her frantic attempts at diversion failed and her depression got worse. I really worried about her.

CAUSES OF DEPRESSION

One of the major causes of depression is metabolism, the physiochemical changes in living organisms. Simply put, some people have a different brain chemistry than others.

In his book *Feeling Good: The New Mood Therapy*, author David D. Burns, MD, explains that some mood disorders run in families. Children may inherit this tendency. He also notes that some of the drugs used to treat high blood pressure seemed to prompt depression in people who are "predisposed to mood disorders."

Environment also plays a role in depression. Many patients in the late stages of Alzheimer's are moved to nursing homes because they need professional care. The patient is forced to leave the comforts of home. By itself, this is a hard adjustment, and the patient may also have to adjust to a different climate.

Leaving Florida was hard for Mom, who had gotten used to the warm temperatures and an outdoor lifestyle. Moving to Minnesota made her very angry.

Although Mom watched weather forecasts on television, she didn't connect them with "real" weather. From the snug warmth of her apartment, a bone-chilling winter day looked like a cozy Christmas card. One morning she called and asked me to drive her to the grocery store. "We shouldn't go out," I said. "It's sleeting, and five to six inches of snow are predicted. I'll take you grocery shopping tomorrow."

"I want to go today," Mom insisted.

"Are you short of food?" I asked.

"No, but I want to go grocery shopping."

Arguing wasn't getting us anywhere, so I agreed to take Mom to the store with our four-wheel drive car. The drive to the store was short, but I could tell the weather was getting worse. Ice was building up on the corners of the windshield, and the wipers made squeaky, shuddering noises on the glass.

Needles of sleet pricked our faces when we got out of the car. We were in the store about fifteen minutes. As we walked to the car Mom exclaimed, "I don't know why anybody would go out today. This weather is awful. I want to go home!" I had to hold my lips together to keep from saying something unkind.

"Down Florida, it's sunny," Mom continued. "Up here, it's dark." Mom had a point. We hadn't seen sunshine for a week, and the bleak midwinter days were hard to endure. I wondered if Mom had Seasonal Affective Disorder (SAD), which is widespread in the Northern Hemisphere.

Seasonal Affective Disorder

If you haven't heard of Seasonal Affective Disorder, it may sound funny to you. But *Minneapolis Star Tribune* writer Tom Majeski says SAD is no joke. It can lead to clinical depression and suicide. Symptoms of the disorder include overeating, a change in sleeping patterns, general fatigue, irritability, less sociability, food cravings, and lower productivity.

Majeski describes light therapy, a professionally supervised treatment for SAD. Each day the afflicted person sits in front of full-spectrum fluorescent lights. The lights are supposed to simulate natural sunlight, which stimulates the body's chemistry.

There were plenty of lamps in Mom's apartment, but she often forgot to turn them on. Whenever she took a nap, Mom closed the curtains. Sometimes the curtains stayed closed. I thought the darkness added to Mom's depression, so I kept trying to open them.

"Oh, leave them closed," Mom would say. "I don't care what's going on out there."

Having the curtains closed made every day a day of darkness. No wonder Mom was depressed. No wonder she had trouble telling day from night. Her depressed attitude about life made my caregiving harder.

Diet

Dietitians have known for years that what we eat influences brain chemistry. Author Marilynn Larkin discusses diet in her book *When Someone You Love Has Alzheimer's.* "Insufficient intake of calories and essential nutrients compound the physical deterioration experienced by people with Alzheimer's," she writes.

Alzheimer's patients who eat lots of sugar may experience behavior swings. Larkin says after they've eaten sweets, many patients have times of increased activity, listlessness, and fatigue. Before she was diagnosed with diabetes, Mom used to binge on sweets at lunch, nap all afternoon, get up, and eat a full dinner.

Diet affects brain function. Good nutrition not only nourishes the body, it also nourishes the brain. If the brain doesn't have the right nutrients, it doesn't function properly. I was glad Mom lived in an assisted living community because she would eat a more balanced diet.

The Anger Connection

Anger and depression are often linked together. The Alzheimer's patient may be angry because he or she is confused, confined, or in pain. Frustration can build to the point of catastrophic reaction, the overreaction to common events or things.

In *Feeling Good: The New Mood Therapy,* Dr. David Burns explains his belief that frustration is the result of unmet expectations. While angry people have the right to try to bring reality in line with their personal thinking, Dr. Burns says the approach is impractical and improbable.

Mounting Losses

For the Alzheimer's patient, every day is a day of loss. These cumulative losses add up. Author Katherine L. Karr thinks depression is a natural response to loss, "whether it be a home, a loving relative or spouse, social supports, a familiar lifestyle, self-image, or that special meaning life once had."

Mom sustained all of these losses and paid a psychiatric price for all of them. Her losses included:

➤ The death of her husband;
➤ The death of her friends;
➤ The loss of her home on Long Island;
➤ The loss of belongings (she kept moving to smaller apartments);
➤ The loss of companionship (which happens to widows and widowers);
➤ The loss of community;
➤ The loss of mathematical ability (she prided herself on her mental calculations);
➤ The loss of clear vision (she had one cataract removed);
➤ The loss of bladder control;
➤ The loss of the life she had known.

The Forgetting Factor

Forgetfulness may fuel depression. Mom kept losing her house key, the mailbox key, and her car keys. At first she joked about her forgetfulness. The jokes stopped. She would have new keys made and then lose them.

As it turned out, the new keys were tossed in a pile on a table by the front door. During our infamous moving weekend, Mom lost her mailbox key. My husband found it in the pile and handed it to her. Mom's eyes widened in surprise. The more we talked with her, the more we realized that she didn't recognize keys as keys, let alone their use.

Knowing Mom, I think her forgetfulness made her more depressed. The title of a *Chicago Tribune* article asks, "Is Forgetting a Danger Sign?" Mom may have asked herself this question. The article details memory slips such as losing keys and says forgetfulness can be "worrisome evidence" of the mind's failures.

Mom may have kept track of her mental failures. If she didn't track them consciously, she may have tracked them unconsciously. Despite forgetting my father's name, she searched for him. Were other losses stored in her mind like lost data in a computer? The human mind is the ultimate computer, and we are just beginning to understand it.

"Depression can also result from feelings of helplessness in the face of growing infirmities," writes Katherine L. Karr in *Promises to Keep: The Family's Role in Nursing Home Care.* "In such instances, it helps to talk about and legitimize the feelings rather than minimize them." Family members should be involved in treatment decisions whenever possible.

Worry

Patients in the early stage of Alzheimer's have the intelligence to worry about the future. Worry contributes to depression. Do I have enough money? Where will I live? What will happen to me? We can't eliminate the patient's worries, but we can anticipate the patient's needs.

Karl Menninger, MD, discussed his personal needs in his article "A Declaration of Probable Needs," which was published in the *Menninger Perspective.* The article was excerpted from "A Declaration of Probable Needs: In Dependent Years, This Much, At Least," published in volume 78, number 8, of the June 1980 issue of *Kansas Alumni.* I have reprinted the list with written permission from the Menninger Foundation, Topeka, Kansas.

Dr. Menninger's List of Probable Needs

1. Comfortable (not too soft) bed;
2. Clean linen on that bed, let's say, once a week;
3. Comforter or blanket within reach, all the time;
4. Corporal safety such as fire protection;
5. Commode that is convenient and accessible and private;
6. Chair near the bed and under a reachable reading light of sufficient power;
7. Communication channels to the outside (telephone, radio, daily papers, weekly news magazine, television within sight and hearing);
8. Common creature comforts such as toothbrush, towels, washcloths, basin, pencils, papers, watch;
9. Contacts with certain outsiders;
10. Competent nursing care;
11. Church services regularly;
12. Cooked and uncooked (fresh) food: tasty, attractive, varied;
13. Chest for private belongings and papers.

This is a reasonable list for the patient and the caregiver. Dr. Menninger tells "oldsters" to start making their own list of personal needs. But the Alzheimer's patient not only loses the ability to make a list, he or she loses the list itself.

We can make out the list for the patient. Best of all, we can make sure the patient is comfortable and try to minimize his or her worries. Meeting these needs will help to reassure the patient. Treatment for depression may also help.

TREATMENT

The diagnosis of depression must be made before treatment begins. If the symptoms of depression are the same as the symptoms of Alzheimer's, how do doctors make the diagnosis? The patient is given a battery of tests that separate depression from other mental problems.

Treatment is prescribed after the diagnosis is made. There are two main types of treatment for depression: psychotherapy (individual and group counseling), and antidepressant medication. A third treatment option, shock therapy, is prescribed in some cases. Treating an Alzheimer's patient for depression can be tricky because he or she may already be taking other medications.

Mom was taking blood pressure medicine, daily insulin, vitamins, anti-clotting medication, over-the-counter pain medication, and other medications. According to research, diabetes alters thinking. Mom's medical condition, actually a combination of diseases, may have made her depressed. Her insulin intake had to be adjusted to her weight and food intake. Once her insulin dosage leveled off, Mom seemed to be more upbeat.

A recent study shows that depression doesn't affect the progression of Alzheimer's disease. Oscar L. Lopez, MD, and his colleagues conducted a longitudinal study of patients with probable Alzheimer's who also met depression criteria. Their findings are reported in "Alzheimer's Disease and Depression: Neuropsychological Impairment and Progression of Illness."

Depressed and nondepressed patients were matched on the basis of sex and their scores on the Mini-Mental State Exam. These patients were part of a highly selected group. The researchers note that depression and Alzheimer's disease impair test performance for different reasons. Patients who are depressed have more trouble with immediate recall, according to the researchers.

"Although there are some discrepant opinions regarding when the incidence of depressive symptoms is greatest in the course of Alzheimer's disease, there is consistent agreement that adequate antidepressant therapy improves the mood of patients with Alzheimer's disease who are also depressed," they write.

The authors don't think depression changes the course of Alzheimer's disease. Some family caregivers refuse mental health treatment. Cognitive therapy won't do much for a patient who isn't cognitive. Moreover, a withdrawn patient can hardly participate in group therapy.

Caregivers may also refuse treatment because of the cost. This issue is explored in an *American Medical News* article called "Society Pays Cost for Undertreatment of Depression." The article says that some primary care physicians don't use mental health systems (managed care) because of the cost, a lack of trained providers, or a fear of offending the patient.

Mental Health Resources

In addition to antidepressants and psychotherapy, caregivers have other resources to turn to:

➤ The National Foundation for Depressive Illness, Inc. (NAFDI);

➤ The National Institute of Mental Health;

➤ The National Mental Health Association;

➤ The National Alliance for the Mentally Ill;

➤ The State Alliance for the Mentally Ill;

➤ The Local Alliance for the Mentally Ill;

➤ Your state mental health association;

➤ The Alzheimer's Association;

➤ The American Association of Retired Persons (AARP).

Call the National Foundation for Depressive Illness hotline at 1-800-239-1263 for recorded information on the symptoms and treatment of depression. This number can also put you in touch with physicians who specialize in the diagnosis and treatment of depression.

Caregiving Tips

Experts have many suggestions on how to take care of a depressed Alzheimer's patient. As helpful as these suggestions are, you must tailor your caregiving to the patient. Marilyn Larkin, the author of *When Someone You Love Has Alzheimer's,* offers the following advice, and I've added some personal comments.

Keep communication lines open. I keep trying to talk with Mom even though she rarely speaks. Who knows what she understands?

Forego pep talks and false hopes. Experts say a calm and compassionate approach works best. Not only does a pep talk anger the patient, it may also set him or her up for more depression.

Promote exercise. As neurotransmitters shut down, coordination becomes more difficult, and the patient gets less exercise. We need to promote exercise because it counteracts depression.

Encourage socialization. If the patient is interested in something, he or she is less apt to be depressed. The patient has a reason to get up in the morning.

Visualization. This suggestion works best in the early stages of the disease. Patients in the later stages may not be able to picture things in their minds.

Discourage alcohol use. Alcohol abuse in the elderly has become a major public health problem. Caregivers need to be aware of this problem and watch for signs of alcohol abuse.

I learned most of these tips by experience. However, I missed one and made the mistake of giving Mom a pep talk. During the talk, I listed all of the things she should be happy about: her attractive apartment, the retirement community services, living close to our family, and contact with her great grandchildren. The pep talk made Mom furious, and I only made this mistake once.

Caregivers need to help depressed people talk about their losses, according to experts. After my disastrous pep talk, I encouraged Mom to talk about the losses in her life, especially her relationship with my father. Talking about my father's alcoholism was upsetting and freeing.

She said living with my father had been difficult and recalled her efforts to get him to stop drinking. "I gave him a choice. He could have a family or the bottle. Your father quit just like that," she said with a snap of her fingers. "We had fun after that, and then he died."

Carol Wolfe Konek talks about her mother's depression in her book, *Daddyboy: A Memoir.* She describes a frightening phone conversation with her mother. Because she had been depressed herself in the past, Konek recognized her mother's depression and told her mother she was probably depressed. The conversation upset her mother.

"You're clinically depressed," she said. She pointed out that her mother slept too much, had no energy, and had limited interests. "You have nothing to look forward to. You do not feel much for other people. Your emotions are flattened," she said. Watching her mother's behavior disturbed Konek.

THE EFFECTS OF DEPRESSION ON CAREGIVERS

The patient's depression may precipitate the caregiver's depression. Each caregiver is affected differently and to a different degree.

A professional caregiver may have a more controlled response to the patient's depression. A spousal caregiver may feel totally lost. Several things may happen when depression and Alzheimer's strike simultaneously. One thing is sure—caregiving takes more time.

The patient's depression may also affect the Alzheimer's

caregiver in other ways:
> ➤ The caregiver may worry more about the patient;
> ➤ The caregiver may be repelled by the patient's verbal or physical aggression;
> ➤ The caregiver may mirror the patient's moods;
> ➤ The caregiver may lose patience;
> ➤ The caregiver may become exhausted.

It's hard to stay upbeat in the company of a depressed person. All of the caregivers I've talked with say the experience is depressing. "I don't know how long I'll be able to do this," one said. Some caregivers worry about "catching" depression from the patient.

"Catching" Depression

If you've ever lived with a depressed person, you know what it feels like. The patient may complain, yell, hit, throw things, accuse, or act out, and yet the caregiver has to be calm and cheerful. Depression may affect spousal caregivers more than others.

Depression isn't a virus—you can't catch it from the Alzheimer's patient. However, you may get so discouraged that you develop situational depression—a psychiatric response to life events. That's why this book ends with a chapter on self-care.

Now that she is vegetative, I can't tell if Mom is depressed. Mom sleeps a lot and eats a little. Sometimes (and the occasions are getting fewer), she is aware of visitors. I suspect that if the patient lives long enough, the brain doesn't have the capacity to generate depressed thoughts.

Many Alzheimer's patients suffer from depression. The caregiver has two complex diseases to deal with—a double duty. Awareness is the first step in treating depression. These action steps will help you tend the patient's body and mind.

What Can You Do?

Become familiar with the progression of depression: the blues, black feelings, and hopelessness.

Become familiar with the symptoms of depression.

Keep a list of the symptoms you observe, including Seasonal Affective Disorder.

Check with the patient's doctor about the medications he or she is taking and their influence on depression.

Make sure the patient eats a balanced diet.

Encourage exercise.

Encourage participation in social activities.

Discourage alcohol use and watch for signs of abuse.

Involve the family in treatment decisions.

Keep communication lines open.

Forego pep talks and false hope.

Remember, you can't make the patient happy; you can only make him or her comfortable.

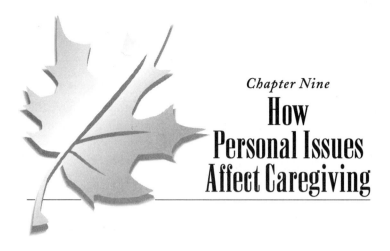

Chapter Nine

How Personal Issues Affect Caregiving

It's a fact—personal issues affect our caregiving.

Ten issues, each of them complex and far-reaching, are examined in this chapter. (You may have other personal issues that you want to add to the list.) The issues are:

➤ Your relationship with the patient;
➤ Your support network;
➤ The language barrier;
➤ Your physical health;
➤ Your mental health;
➤ Unresolved grief;
➤ Grief clusters;
➤ Stress;
➤ Sandwich Generation;
➤ Not enough time.

YOUR RELATIONSHIP WITH THE PATIENT

All of the issues are important, although your relationship with the patient may well be the foundation of caregiving. After watching professional caregivers in action, I've decided many have a natural aptitude for it. Maybe you do, too.

One such "natural" caregiver works in Mom's nursing home. She is blonde, bubbly, and always cheerful. Despite nasty weather and her own problems, she acts the same. Her patience is limitless and her kindness is humbling.

I think the retirement community is fortunate to have this caregiver on the staff. The best thing about her, the most important thing, is that she loves her job. All caregivers would enjoy what they do in an ideal world.

All too often, however, professional caregivers don't like their work or work conditions. The wages may be low; the hours may be long; the facility may be crowded and dreary. Professional caregivers change jobs for a variety of reasons.

Some facilities have what Marilynn Larkin calls a "revolving door" staff. In her book *When Someone You Love Has Alzheimer's,* Larkin tells family members to be wary of a facility that is constantly hiring new people.

The "revolving door" is one indication of a caregiver's unhappiness. A sour expression may be another. Daily conversation also gives us clues to the caregiver's state of happiness. Here are some actual comments from family caregivers:

➤ "All she does is criticize. I never do anything right."
➤ "He thinks I want his money."
➤ "Every time we get ready to leave town, she has a health crisis. We're prisoners."
➤ "My mother and I never got along and we never will."
➤ "We fight like cats and dogs."
➤ "I don't have a life any more."

Despite comments like these, love blooms amidst the thorns of anger. These family caregivers love their parents. So what's the problem? The problem may be a leftover parent-child relationship. According to Judith Viorst, author of *Necessary Losses,* troubled and wholesome families often assign roles to family members. You may be the responsible child, the middle child, or the family clown. Being a caregiver may alter your role. "In building lives of our own, we challenge our family's myths and roles—and, of course, we challenge the rigid rules of childhood," she writes.

Just because you're an adult doesn't mean you have forgotten your childhood role. Although you are a responsible caregiver, you may find yourself falling back into those roles. Mom and I had a wonderful mother-daughter relationship, and I can't remember ever arguing with her.

I find comfort in this relationship today. No matter what happens, I can remember our loving and respectful relationship—mother and daughter.

YOUR SUPPORT NETWORK

During the last two years I've had many trying days—days when I knew I needed help, and asked for it. But some caregivers have an "I'll do this myself" attitude. Either they are ashamed to ask for help, blind to the need for help, or unaware of support services. While this is a confident approach to caregiving, it can also be harmful.

Barbara W. McCabe RN, PhD, and her colleagues discuss support networks in their article "Availability and Utilization of Services by Alzheimer's Disease Caregivers." They say rural communities have more tight-knit support systems than urban communities have.

According to the researchers, rural communities also have fewer support services. To learn more about the influence of demographics on the use of support services, they conducted a study.

Questionnaires were sent to 212 Nebraska residents who received an Alzheimer's newsletter. One hundred nineteen of the questionnaires were returned, and eleven of these were blank. Respondents were asked to answer questions about their use of support services in relation to the Alzheimer's patient. A statistical analysis of the data was conducted.

One finding: 65 percent of the respondents had no support services other than nursing homes and support groups.

The researchers also learned that some caregivers didn't use support services because they didn't know about them. Despite the fact that more services were offered in urban areas, family caregivers who lived in rural areas used more services overall.

The researchers think many family caregivers provide care at the risk of their own health. All caregivers need help. We can't do this alone. But when caregivers try to tap into community support systems, many find confusing and fragmented services. They may also run into language barriers.

THE LANGUAGE BARRIER

Older caregivers turn to family, friends, and the church for support. Where do younger caregivers turn? Cathleen M. Connell, PhD, and her colleagues examine support systems in their article, "Increasing Coordination of the Dementia Service Delivery Network: Planning for the Community Outreach Education Program."

Caregivers encounter many barriers, say the researchers, including dated information, poor coordination of services, and lack of professional skills. The caregivers who are members of minority groups avoid formal support systems because of cultural and language barriers. It's hard to trust someone you don't understand or who doesn't understand you.

There's another barrier, too, and that's staffing. "Access problems are further complicated by the limited number of minority health professionals who provide specialized services, especially in low-income neighborhoods," note the researchers.

Their solution is a community-based support network. The Community Outreach Education Program was created to serve Michigan health professionals, service providers, local organizations, and families. The article details plans for this network. Although no results are reported, the authors plan to use questionnaires, site visits, and meetings with community contacts to evaluate the network.

Few communities have this kind of support. Is a poor support network better than nothing? Only the caregiver can decide. The Alzheimer's Association slogan, "Someone to Stand by You," is a good one to keep in mind. Surely the caregivers who have health problems need someone to stand by them.

YOUR PHYSICAL HEALTH

The caregiver's physical health affects his or her daily performance. One caregiver needed major surgery. In order to have this surgery she had to get a sitter for her husband—an added cost not covered by medical insurance. Plus, older caregivers don't bounce back as quickly as they used to.

Brenda F. Bergman-Evans, RNC, PhD, focuses on spousal caregivers in her article "Alzheimer's and Related Disorders: Loneliness, Depression, and Social Support of Spousal Caregivers." Citing previous research, she says spousal caregivers "have a higher than expected rate of diabetes, arthritis, ulcers, and anemia, as well as poorer health perceptions…fewer doctor visits than the general population."

Having a yearly physical isn't a choice for me; it's a necessity. An eye exam is part of the physical. I've already had laser surgery in one eye for a detaching retina, and my other eye is starting to show the same symptoms. So ophthalmologists are monitoring me closely.

If you discount the normal effects of aging, I'm in good health. Health issues seem to be more important now that I'm a grandmother. I eat a low-fat, low-salt diet, and I exercise a half hour every day. This is the busiest, most challenging time of my life. While I love the challenges, I'm also more tired at the end of a day. No late night television for me—I'm in bed at 9:30 P.M. and up with the birds.

YOUR MENTAL HEALTH

All caregivers have times when they feel mentally fatigued. The never-ending demands of caregiving take their toll. Although I'm willing to accept responsibility, Mom has suffered from dementia for fourteen years, and I'm getting tired.

It's also not unusual for a professional caregiver to be a family caregiver. Susan K. Theut, MD, MPH, discusses her dual roles of daughter and caregiver in her article "Caregiver's Anticipatory Grief in Dementia: A Pilot Study." Theut says the spouses of demented patients feel anger, guilt, anxiety, depression, and loss. The family caregiver may not be able to distance himself or herself from a loved one. The professional caregiver may tire of watching the constant decline and death of patients. Theut experienced both roles. Who can keep up with these feelings?

Nobody. That's why support groups exist. The Mayo Clinic Alzheimer's Disease Center runs "regular" and special support groups, cosponsored by the Alzheimer's Association of Minnesota. Two special groups, one for daughters and one for male caregivers, were started to meet caregivers' needs. Weekly dementia education classes are also offered. The classes are free, and no registration is required.

Support groups offer practical information and a sense of kinship. Joining a group can give you a chance to de-stress. But the family caregivers who struggle with unresolved grief may continue to feel stressed. Unresolved grief is a powerful emotion.

UNRESOLVED GRIEF

Researchers say it's difficult to evaluate the impact of unresolved grief. Pamela N. Enlow, MSN, RN, describes her grief in "Coping With Anticipatory Grief." Although she writes about herself, she could have been writing about me.

Enlow tells how she prepared for her mother's death three

times. She prayed for the release of her mother's soul. Despite her emotional pain, anticipatory grief promised resolution for Enlow, an ending to her mother's life story. The ending wasn't forthcoming.

She writes, "My mother lives, lives on in a nursing home, debilitated, unable to walk, unable to talk coherently, mentally confused…This daughter could handle the death of her beloved mother, but this living death, the loss of mother as I once knew her is a loss that leaves grief unresolved."

Watching a loved one slowly die is a constant anguish. Edward Myers discusses this kind of anguish in his book *When Parents Die: A Guide for Adults.* According to Myers, successive illnesses such as kidney damage and cardiac arrhythmias make the burden heavier."A long illness lacks the sheer shock effect of a sudden death," he explains, "but it can nevertheless cause tremendous strain."

Myers says the strain of caregiving comes from role reversal, being a member of the sandwich generation, and "double binds." While taking care of a failing parent you may be neglecting your partner, your kids, your job, your community, your church, or yourself. As Myers explains, "It's impossible to do anything without getting into a fix."

He's right. When I get up in the morning, I wonder if this will be the day I get The Phone Call. I'm expecting the news of Mom's death and dreading this news. Words fascinate me and, because I'm a word person, I wonder what Mom's last words will be.

Maybe her last words will be, "I want to go shopping." Her last words may be, "Thanks for everything," a poignant reminder of our Sunday night suppers. She may resort to her favorite refrain, "I'm A.A.A. Alive, alert, and alluring!" The mother of my childhood had been quick with words.

In February of 1997, Mom celebrated her ninety-third birthday. I gave her a pink cyclamen, bursting with full blooms and buds. Mom reached toward the flowers and said, "They're pretty." Would these be her last words? They might be.

I've visited her since then and she hasn't said anything. Mom has lost so much weight I hardly know her. This really is a living death for her and a constant strain for me. Unresolved grief is part of my day and "normal" grief awaits me.

Senator Jay Rockefeller talked about his grief on the CNN television special, "Alzheimer's: The Long Good Bye." With raw emotion he spoke of his mother's death. He also explained his appearance on the program. "I wanted people to know how horrible her death was ... and I think, I think it is the worst way to die."

Family caregivers can be paralyzed by unresolved grief. The symptoms include sadness, crying spells, impatience, nervousness, anxiety, anger, depression, and loss of hope. If you have many of these symptoms or are overcome with grief, you might want to contact a grief counselor.

GRIEF CLUSTERS

At this time of life, family caregivers are starting to see their loved ones die. So many of our friends have died that I keep a supply of sympathy cards on hand. None of us can predict life, and we certainly can't predict grief clusters, a confluence of events that cause grief.

Remember that grief is a response to change. Grief clusters sap our energy and muddle our minds. The family may be forced to move. Grown children may need the caregiver's help. Friends may die within months of each other. I went through many changes in a relatively short period of time, and they all made me grieve.

➤ I cried when we moved out of our dream house.
➤ I cried when my dearest friend moved away.
➤ I cried when our daughter went through a painful divorce.

➤ I cried after our granddaughter called to say, in a hesitant voice, "Daddy's gone."

➤ I cried when a friend died.

➤ I cried when another friend died a few months later.

Bettyclare Moffatt writes about grief clusters in her book *Soulwork: Clearing the Mind, Opening the Heart, Replenishing the Spirit.* When life tests us, Moffatt says, we may be able to function, survive, and still suppress our grief.

"Sometimes we heal a little or a lot, but never fully," she explains. "Another crisis comes. Another loved one is ill. Someone else dies and someone else. Love walks away from us. The places where we once flourished fall into ruin."

STRESS

Crisis leads to stress. Family caregivers start to feel stress in the early stages of Alzheimer's. Stress can build until it goes off the "stress meter." Brenda F. Bergman-Evans, RNC, PhD, examines stress in her article "Alzheimer's and Related Disorders: Loneliness, Depression, and Social Support of Spousal Caregivers." Despite all of the research that's been done, "little is known about the effect of institutional placement on caregiver stress," says Bergman-Evans. Spousal stress often begins when family members first hear the diagnosis of probable Alzheimer's disease.

Poor understanding of the nature and progress of the disease also contributes to stress. Family members who deny the illness feel stressed. Bergman-Evans says there's also a "deep sense of loss and sadness as the disease progresses." A spousal caregiver may feel guilty (another kind of stress) for putting a loved one in a nursing home.

After visiting their loved one, many spouses go home to an empty house. The quiet is stressful. Bergman-Evans writes, "Loss of the companionship of their significant other, forced social isolation, increased responsibility, and the increased emotional burden of caregiving may individually or mutually predispose the spousal caregiver to feelings of loneliness."

Prolonged grief is a major stressor for family caregivers. Robert Fulton, PhD, and Robert Bendiksen, PhD, discuss prolonged grief in their book *Death & Identity*. They explain, "The stress, both physical and emotional, of a long grieving over an expected loss may take a terrible toll on the individual."

You may not realize the toll you're paying. In fact, you may not know you're stressed. According to Edward Myers, the author of *When Parents Die: A Guide for Adults*, stress can be a subliminal feeling. It can stay hidden for a time and then take you by surprise. Myers thinks the long haul of caregiving "will disrupt most families."

Once you're feeling stressed it's hard to de-stress. At least, that's been my experience. I tried to pinpoint the stressors in my life. What could I do about them? Here are some of my stressors and some possible solutions.

Stressor	Solution
Mom's paperwork	Do a little each day
State and federal income taxes	Hire a professional tax service
Shopping for Mom	Buy extra socks, underwear, etc., when I go shopping
Time involved in caregiving	Daily self-care
Mom's anger and combativeness	Focus on the cause, not the behavior
Dwindling funds	Get a financial aid form and start filling it out

Having more than one family member with dementia is another stressor. Some families have two parents with probable Alzheimer's disease. Now that's stress!

THE SANDWICH GENERATION

Being a member of the sandwich generation is another stressor. I think *sandwich generation* is a mild term for the realities of caregiving. My caregiving isn't decreasing, it's increasing, and I'm constantly torn. Who needs me most— my children, my grandchildren, my mother, or my husband?

Lately, it's been my husband; for on a beautiful May morning, when the air was soft and the sun was bright, my husband's aorta split in two.

The dissection happened on the way to work. My husband was driving past the hospital when he felt a sharp pain in his back. "It felt like somebody had stabbed me," he later recalled. He thought he might be having muscle spasms, a side effect of his blood pressure medicine.

As the pain increased, my husband recalled a recent X-ray that showed a slight change in his aorta. Fearing the worst, he headed for the hospital emergency room. A new parking ramp was under construction and equipment hid the entrance from his view. So he went around the block again.

By now the pain was acute and sweat was running down his face. He parked the car near the entrance. A workman saw him and rushed inside to get the response team. These three things—the workman's help, my husband's lead, and the team's skill—saved his life.

But would he survive?

In the intensive care unit, he looked more dead than alive. I thought I was going to be a widow. After I visited my husband, I visited my mother. The days blurred in my mind. How long could I keep this up? To conserve energy, I stopped visiting Mom and focused on my husband.

My husband had the type of dissection that can be treated with medicine, not surgery, and doctors said he was doing well. I read by his bedside while he slept. When I was at the hospital, I appeared to be strong, but when I got home, I cried like a baby.

One night my father-in-law called to check on my husband's condition. I updated him and said, "I'm going to hang up now, Dad. I have to cry for about two hours."

After lots of thought (and lots of tissues), I came to some decisions. First, I decided to let myself cry in public. After all, I was grieving for two people. Second, I knew I had to take care of myself, so I vowed to eat balanced meals. Third, I decided to find strength in thirty-nine years of marriage and the love my husband and I shared.

Although these decisions helped me to plan, they didn't change my "membership" in the sandwich generation. I was very worried about the twins. Grandpa had become an important person in their lives—the person who read to them, showed them the attic (exciting stuff), demonstrated tools, and built them a seesaw. His illness would upset them.

My daughter decided to tell the twins the truth. Since they couldn't understand the concept of a dissected aorta, she told them that Grandpa had a broken heart. She took them to the hospital so they could see, for themselves, how he was doing. A nurse described their visit to me that afternoon.

"How did the twins respond?" I asked.

"They were adorable, just like Raggedy Ann and Andy," she said. "They stood in his room, looked at him with big eyes, and never said a word." Visiting Grandpa was just what the twins needed, and he needed them.

After ten days in intensive care my husband came home. My daughter and the twins visited him almost every day. They watched Grandpa's condition go from lying on the couch, to sitting up, to walking. "Seeing the twins made me feel better," my husband said.

Jo Horne has some advice for the sandwich generation in her book *Caregiving: Helping an Aging Loved One*. The caregiver's children need to know that their lives are going to change, Horne says, and that all family members may be asked to make sacrifices. I also think family members need to know about the time crunch.

NOT ENOUGH TIME

Time is a major sacrifice for many caregivers, especially since time can't be regained. Many spousal caregivers are virtually confined to their homes. Family caregivers may run themselves ragged as they try to care for parents and adult children. Caregiving has a bright, hopeful side and a dark, discouraging side.

Anne Boykin, PhD, RN, and Jill Winland-Brown, EdD, RN, talk about time in their article "The Dark Side of Caring: Challenges of Caregiving." They think the "subtleness of the progression of Alzheimer's disease" forces caregivers into giving more time and energy.

I'm pretty good at time management, but caregiving threw my plans off kilter. There was too much to do and too little time to do it. Although I made lists and prioritized them, the time crunch got to me. Edward Myers discusses the time crunch in his book *When Parents Die.*

"The problem is that many of the obligations involved, although not mutually exclusive, end up competing for time and attention," he writes. "It isn't just that 'there are only so many hours in a day.' There is also only so much emotional energy, only so much patience, only so much self-confidence."

But there's another facet to the time issue. Not one of the countless medical articles I've read said time gets more precious as you get older. As my brother explained, "The hourglass of my life is nearly empty, and I'm counting every grain of sand."

I, too, am counting grains of sand. In the middle of the night, I wonder how many years I have left. What books will I write? Will I have dementia like Mom? Will our children be taking care of me? Questions like these help me to appreciate life. I don't take it for granted any more.

OTHER ISSUES

Each of the issues I've discussed affected my caregiving. Two other issues also played a part. I didn't put them on the list because they might not apply to you. On second thought, maybe they do.

Adult Children of Alcoholics

There are thousands, if not millions, of adult children of alcoholics in our country and I'm one of them. According to researcher and writer Janet Geringer Woititz, EdD, the adult children of alcoholics usually have thirteen characteristics. She discusses these characteristics in her book *Adult Children of Alcoholics.*

Although I don't have all of the characteristics, I have two that apply to my caregiving situation. Often I judge myself without mercy, and I'm overly responsible. If you're in trouble, I'll be there—the durable, dependable friend. Because I'm the adult child of an alcoholic, I always want to fix things.

I can't fix my mother. Every day I feel more helpless. I know I'm helping by managing her finances, paying her bills, buying the things she needs, and visiting her. Yet this isn't enough, in my mind. I keep wondering if there's more I could do.

The Patient's Delusions

Over time, Mom's old delusions—that Dad was coming to get her and that my brother was remarrying his former wife—were replaced by new ones. The new delusions became the focus of her life. I had no idea these delusions would cause so much trouble.

One delusion involved returning to Long Island and moving in with a friend. I think the friend died years ago, but Mom was sure her friend was expecting her. The delusion became Mom's escape plan, something that would get her out of nursing care. She kept asking, "When am I going to Long Island?"

The other delusion was that my brother was coming to visit. Actually, the delusion was based on a partial truth. Several times my brother and his wife had come from Florida to visit Mom. But she forgot their visits in less than two hours.

"What time is he coming?" Mom would ask. "Is he going to stay with you?"

I tried not to answer Mom's questions because I wanted to avoid conflict. However, the silence strategy didn't work. Mom kept harping and harping until I answered her. To make matters worse, she forgot my brother had remarried and thought his new wife (a marvelous addition to our family) worked in nursing care.

I finally told Mom the truth about my brother. "He was already here," I said.

"No, no, he's coming today," Mom would insist.

"He was here and he's gone back to Florida," I would reply.

"Why would he say he was coming if he wasn't coming to visit me?" she would ask. "He wouldn't do that."

I watched the delusions evolve. Each started with a false idea. The idea would increase in frequency. Then Mom would convince herself that the delusion was true. When the delusion didn't come true, I became the target of her anger. If you were to diagram a delusion, it would look something like this:

1. Misperception (initial delusion).
2. Increase in frequency.
3. Conviction that delusion is true.
4. Disappointment.
5. Anger and conflict.

Mom decided I was lying to her and plotting against her. I tried to avoid arguments. "I love you. I've told you the truth. I'm not going to argue with you," became my standard reply. The delusions lasted until Mom lost the ability to create meaningful sentences. Now that she rarely speaks, I don't know what she is thinking.

Many personal issues affect our caregiving. These issues don't have to be weaknesses; they can become our strengths. Personal issues tie us together like the colorful threads of a tapestry. These issues can enrich our lives and the lives of patients. We are not alone. Hand-in-hand, we strive to give Alzheimer's patients good care and take care of ourselves at the same time. There are many insights we can share.

What Can You Do?

Identify the personal issues that affect your caregiving.

Examine your relationship with the patient. What are the strengths? What are the weaknesses?

Research available support services.

Accept help willingly.

Navigate and negotiate the barriers you encounter.

Take care of your body.

Take care of your mind.

Be aware of the symptoms of unresolved grief.

Learn how to de-stress yourself.

Learn time-management techniques.

Think about the influence of your background and family role on caregiving.

Approach delusions with kindness and compassion.

Think of your personal issues as strengths.

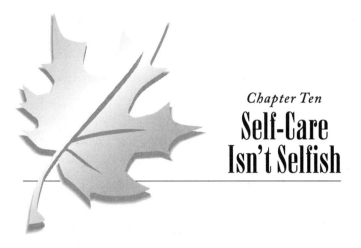

Self-Care Isn't Selfish

So far we've been talking about care of the Alzheimer's patient. Now it's time to think about taking care of you—the caregiver. Self-care is a vital component of patient care. Eric B. Larson, MD, MPH, makes this point in his editorial, "Alzheimer's Disease in the Community."

He writes, "Until we have an effective treatment for Alzheimer's disease, the best strategy is to assist actively patients, families, and caregivers with the long-term management of the problems associated with the disease." While this strategy is becoming reality, the reality is slow in coming.

Many caregivers take self-care for granted. They think self-care is automatic, something that happens in between their caregiving tasks. Self-care isn't automatic—it's a conscious, adaptive process that changes with time.

CASE FOR SELF-CARE

Too many caregivers feel adrift and alone. Karen S. Peterson talks about the mental and physical costs of caregiving in her *USA Today* article "More Spend Time Caring for Elders." Citing a survey of American Association of Retired Persons (AARP), Peterson says more than forty million households in the U.S. provide at least forty hours of care each week.

In addition, some 1.6 million households provide twenty to forty hours of care each week. Peterson also cites the

National Alliance for Caregiving (NAC), which states that caregivers are usually women. Families that are involved in caregiving spend two billion out-of-pocket dollars in the process. Many caregivers go without and sacrifice their needs for the needs of the patient.

The caregiver may also go without a self-care plan. You may think you're practicing self-care and spend little time on it. Even if you have a self-care plan, it may be a cobbled one, hastily put together. There are distinct advantages to having a self-care plan:

➤ You think things through ahead of time.
➤ You have a framework of support.
➤ You are better prepared for emergencies.
➤ You lead a more balanced life.
➤ You have a happier, healthier life.
➤ You can adapt the plan as needed.

Without a self-care plan, the caregiver runs out of energy. Some caregivers have become martyrs to the cause. Once you have given in to this kind of thinking, it's hard to turn your thinking around. Experts say that caregivers should avoid the martyr trap. Are you a martyr?

THE MARTYR TRAP

A Parke-Davis book, *Caring for the Caregiver,* defines martyrs as caregivers who put aside their own needs and expend all of their energy on the Alzheimer's patient. Pride and poor information may cause the caregiver to refuse help. "One day these people may collapse under the strain," note the authors.

Even if you did not consciously decide to be a martyr, you may still be one. The result is the same. Instead of one person in need of help—the Alzheimer's patient—now there are two. Becoming a martyr not only misdirects your energy, it can turn you into a bitter, exhausted person.

According to the authors of *Caring for the Caregiver,* the

wisest thing you can do "is to stay mentally and physically strong." This is easier said than done.

FEMALE CAREGIVERS

The eldest and/or unmarried daughter is designated as the family caregiver in some cultures. Her task is to take care of her aging parents. Because they have been trained for the role since birth, these females accept it. An only daughter may be designated as the family caregiver in much the same way.

In our own culture, many women have given up their careers in order to be family caregivers. Unfortunately, what sounds like a good idea at the beginning often turns into a life of bitterness. These caregivers may dedicate ten, fifteen, or more years to the patient. For them, there is no light at the end of the tunnel.

"Everyone asks about my husband," one caregiver said. "What about me? How am I doing?"

MALE CAREGIVERS

The demand for caregivers seems to exceed the supply. As more males become caregivers, they are discovering, like their female counterparts, that caregiving is open-ended. The realities of dementia are far-reaching and, at times, shocking.

Like female caregivers, some male caregivers think self-care is selfish. Nothing could be farther from the truth. Self-care isn't selfish; it is necessary for the caregiver's survival. This deliberate process includes the care of body, mind, and soul.

TAKING CARE OF YOUR BODY

Alzheimer's disease changes both the patient and the caregiver. The caregiver's health may suffer during the course of the disease. Author Carol Wolfe Konek describes her mother's caregiving in her book, *Daddyboy: A Memoir.* At the time of Konek's writing, her mother lived in California, "trapped in a house with a dead man in a live body." Konek tells how her mother rages against this fact of life. As she watches her mother care for her father, Konek sees that her mother has become old and is no longer the "tough, sturdy woman" of her childhood. Now her mother is weak and more confused.

Many caregivers lack the resilience of youth. That's why we need regular physicals, regular exercise, and a balanced diet. Caregiving requires lots of energy, and we must take care of ourselves if we're going to do it. We can also find ways to be more efficient.

Review your caregiving tasks. Can you do something another way? Can any tasks be combined? Will a change of sequence help? Build some "me time" into the day while you're reviewing your caregiving tasks. If you don't do this, you'll only become more stressed.

Caregivers often think of stress as a mental condition, although it has many physical symptoms: overeating, poor appetite, sleep problems, headaches, backaches, more colds and flu, and fatigue. What good are you to the patient if you're sick? Not much. And, you not only need to take care of your physical health—you need to take care of your mental health as well.

TAKING CARE OF YOUR MIND
An "interior clean-up" is a way of taking care of your mind. Bettyclare Moffatt tells how to go about it in her book *Soulwork: Clearing the Mind, Opening the Heart, Replenishing the Spirit*. She recommends an interior clean-up "when joy is covered and clouded over by too much stuff." Moffatt says the mental exercise has three basic steps.

First, you clear your mind of mental garbage—things such as old resentments and buried feelings. Next, you put this garbage in imaginary trash bags and throw them out.

(Moffatt even puts her mental garbage bags out on an imaginary curb.) Last, you replace your mental garbage with creativity and humor. Repeat the exercise when necessary.

Although I didn't have any old resentments against my mother, I was carrying around some mental garbage, including the notion that Mom would suddenly brighten up. I knew this was denial, and yet I couldn't get rid of the idea.

The idea surfaced just before Thanksgiving. Despite her severe dementia, I thought Mom could come to our family dinner. It would take two of us to get her out of the car and into the house. She would sit in the rocking chair, sip a diluted glass of wine, and watch the twins play. I mentioned the idea to the director of nursing.

"I don't know if Mom could come for Thanksgiving," I began tentatively. "She's failing fast but..." The look on the director's face stopped me cold.

"Not this year," she said. "She needs to be here with us."

I nodded my head in agreement. Mom would never come to dinner again. So we had Thanksgiving without her. As had become our custom, we held hands around the table and said, "God bless us every one." In my mind I blessed my mother.

All through dinner, however, I kept imagining that Mom would arrive. My husband would open the back door, I'd hear the little ping of the hinges, and he'd help Mom up the steps.

"Sorry we're late," he would say.

"You dinner smells delicious," Mom would say, nibbling pieces of turkey and stuffing. "Remember, I have to have a corner seat because I'm left-handed."

Instead, I smiled and talked and held back my tears. My sadness was quickly replaced with reason. Coming for dinner had become a threatening experience for Mom, a foray into alien territory. Mom didn't know who we were, where she was, or how to act.

Besides, Mom *was* at our Thanksgiving table. I could see her in the faces of our daughters, I could hear her in the giggles of our grandchildren. Mom's values had been imprinted in my mind, and she will always be a part of me. I knew that if I did nothing else in life, I would pass these values on to the next generation.

Self-Care Through Dementia Education

In many communities, dementia education has become part of adult education. The Mayo Clinic Alzheimer's Disease Center, for example, has weekly dementia education sessions. The topics include genetics, sundowning and shadowing, patient needs, and others.

Staff writer Warren Wolfe details a dementia workshop in his *Minneapolis Star Tribune* article "Helping Dad by Helping Themselves." The workshop was funded by a grant from the National Institutes of Health. Thirty-two families have participated in the seven-week program so far. Those families are being compared with families in a control group, who were not enrolled in the program.

Standardized tests were given before and after the workshop. During that time, the control group families felt their caregiving burden had risen, whereas the workshop families thought their family problems had fallen. Clearly, more families need to become involved in this kind of training. As Wolfe says, "Without significant help from other relatives, the primary care giver often just runs out of energy."

His article includes comments from caregivers. One caregiver realized he had been pushing his father too hard. Another learned the value of routines. Family caregivers not only learned about Alzheimer's, they also learned how to pull together. This may be the most significant outcome of the workshop.

COMPUTER NETWORK SUPPORT

Other caregivers are turning to computer networks for support. Robert L. Gallienne, BA, RN, ND, and his colleagues discuss these networks in "Alzheimer's Caregivers: Psychosocial Support via Computer Networks."

"Family members may be struggling with finding meaning in their loved one's suffering and thus need spiritual support and guidance," the authors explain. They also say that caregivers need information about support services, home care, and self-care.

Technology has come to the rescue with ComputerLink, designed explicitly for caregivers. It started with homebound caregivers and expanded to a subnetwork on the Cleveland, Ohio, public access network. Forty-seven caregivers who had participated in an Alzheimer's study, had access to a private mail system and a bulletin board. Both were twenty-four-hour services. The authors think the twenty-four-hour access is one of the most valuable features of the network. Anonymity is another valuable feature. On-line support was provided by a nurse moderator and peer group members.

Having a nurse on hand turned out to be very important. The nurse was there to "hear" people's needs and respond directly. Traditional support methods aren't necessarily appropriate for all caregivers, say the researchers. They add, "Never before has there been an opportunity for nurses to be so innovative."

Luke Shockman described a family caregiver's computer support in a *Rochester Post-Bulletin* article, "Caring for the Caregiver." The article focuses on Bob Hoffman and his wife, Shirley, who was diagnosed with probable Alzheimer's at age fifty-two. While caring for his wife, Bob became a "prisoner in his own home." So Bob turned to the Internet and the World Wide Web for support. He started his own web site and used it to share personal feelings. I talked to

Bob about the site and how it's changed. "It started out as a personal journal and has grown into general information," he explained. Bob has added article reprints, book reviews, and e-mail excerpts to the site, and he gets mail from around the world. Recently his site was reviewed by a Japanese newspaper. Use http://www.isl.net/~hoffcomp/ to reach Bob and learn more about caregiving. Other support systems are being created to meet the increasing demand for them. Help ranges from handy-man services to neighborly concern. Of course, the neighbors can't help you unless they know you need help. Self-care must be an honest and adaptive process.

SELF-CARE AS A PROCESS

If you're like me, your self-care plan may have gotten off to a slow start. Over time, I realized I would have to do more for myself. I needed a basic self-care plan, something I could turn to when I was feeling down or stressed. Because you have different needs, your self-care plan may be different from mine.

Katherine L. Karr lists some self-care tips in her book *Promises to Keep: The Family's Role in Nursing Home Care.* The suggestions include learning how to spot your stress signals, arranging brief getaways, and enjoying the moment. The question is, *can* you enjoy the moment?

As Edna L. Ballard, ACSW, and Cornelia M. Poer, BA, point out in their book *Sexuality and the Alzheimer's Patient,* you may not enjoy the same interests and hobbies that you used to. "Caregivers may find that things, which gave them pleasure earlier, no longer hold appeal or their attention," they write.

You may have to find new interests. In fact, the authors say you must make the effort to do this. If you're going to continue to be a caregiver, you need to feed your inner self. Ballard and Poer recommend doing things to boost your self-esteem, such as paying attention to your appearance, exercising regularly, and eating right. They also say we should take the time to fix ourselves attractive meals. Not only do these positive behaviors help us to feel better, Ballard and Poer say, they help us to feel less lonely.

THE WHOLE PERSON APPROACH

All of the reading I've done recommends a whole person approach to self-care. Ballard and Poer divide this approach into four groups: maintenance needs, self-actualizing needs, self-esteem needs, and belonging needs. Each group heading is followed by a list of examples.

Maintenance needs include learning to pace yourself. Self-actualizing needs include making a wish list. Self-esteem needs include refusing to give way to "poor me" thinking. Belonging needs include joining a phone hot line.

You may have convinced yourself that the patient's needs *always* come first. This isn't true. Caregivers have needs, too, and you must keep them in mind as you go about your caregiving. Instead of dividing my needs into groups, I simply made a list of the things I need:

➤ More quiet time.

➤ More time with my husband.

➤ Help at home.

➤ Social contacts.

➤ An exercise program.

➤ New interests.

➤ Weekly contact with our grandchildren.

Use the "I Need" form in Appendix D to make your list. Cross out items as your needs are met. Six months from now, you may have a completely different list of needs. Filling out the "I Need" list is also a good way to start your self-care plan.

MAKING A SELF-CARE PLAN

When you make your self-care plan, try not to get bogged down with details. After you think, narrow your plan down to simple phrases or words. I used the words *body, mind,* and *soul* for the framework of my plan. Then I thought of action steps to go with these words. To make your plan:

1. Select key words (or headings);
2. Match action steps to the headings;
3. Try out the plan;
4. Modify the plan as needed;
5. Review your plan regularly.

My self-care plan is a work in progress and I continue to revise it. For example, I realized I needed even more quiet time. Being an Alzheimer's caregiver changes your life. In fact, your life may now be vastly different from the one you have known.

A NEW AND DIFFERENT LIFE

Dartmouth College professor, author, and poet Sheila Harvey Tanzer describes her different life in an article published in *Dartmouth Medicine.* She wrote the article, "In the Wake of Loss," about her husband Lawrence who had been a professor of French and Italian at Dartmouth for many years.

A colleague had called her about the neurological tests her husband had recently taken. The colleague's diagnosis was probable Alzheimer's disease. Sheila focused on the word *probable* because it gave her more room for hope. She writes, "Little did I know that eight years later, the dynamic professor would not recognize his own reflection in the mirror, nor would the gifted linguist, fluent in three languages, be able to utter a single word."

Sheila tells how her husband's memory loss became an invisible wedge between them, driving them progressively apart. "I felt abandoned," she writes, "trapped by an affliction that ruled both our lives."

During this bleak time she drew strength from past conversations with her husband and the writings of psychotherapist Viktor Frankl. She prayed and wrote about her feelings in journal entries, letters, and poems. Rather than focusing on her pain, she focused on her mental freedom. Sheila's children helped her to adjust and adapt to her husband's death. She enrolled in a hospice training program, took courses at a local community college, and started teaching at Dartmouth. Today, she is the wife of Radford Tanzer, MD, and head of the Upper Valley Hostel Board. As she worked to construct a new life from the ashes of despair, Sheila discovered a wellspring of strength inside herself. You may find a similar wellspring.

GROWTH THROUGH PAIN

Every Alzheimer's caregiver has moments of emotional pain. Each moment brings us to a crossroad in life. We can let ourselves be overcome by pain, or we can let ourselves grow from experience. It's a hard choice.

There is no cure for Alzheimer's disease at this time, so you know the outcome. Your best efforts won't save the patient, and he or she will grow more frail, more demented, and more lost to you. I can't believe the physical changes in my mother. Once she was overweight, even for a large-boned person, and now she is virtually skin and bones. Mom is dying cell-by-cell, and the emotional pain is white-hot, searing, and fierce.

I expressed this pain in an odd way by starting to imitate my mother. When I walked upstairs or downstairs, I clutched the railing for support. Despite an excellent lung capacity, I would rest on the stairs halfway up. I did this for several weeks, until I realized what was going on.

Years ago, I had done something similar; I had started dressing like my mother. Finally, our younger daughter took me aside and told me I was dressing at least fifteen years older than my age. As surprising as this news was, I realized she was right, and I got rid of my dowdy clothes.

Acting like Mom was a way of identifying with her. It may also be an expression of anticipatory grief. I know that observing Mom's decline has been one of the most painful experiences of my life. As Katherine L. Karr writes in her book *Promises to Keep: The Family's Role in Nursing Home Care,* "It is important to recognize when you are in a situation where death may be the only final resolution to the emotional and physical pain your family member experiences."

Despite our best efforts, the Alzheimer's patient will grow more fragile and die. Some caregivers face this reality; others go around it or wall themselves in to avoid pain. You can't stay walled in forever.

Writer Alla Bozarth-Campbell believes that pain is an essential ingredient of life. In her book *Life Is Goodbye, Life Is Hello: Grieving Well Through All Kinds of Loss,* she discusses the value of pain. "Pain is an essential part of any growth process—the process of growing up, growing old, growing beyond grief."

Bozarth-Campbell thinks we sabotage ourselves when we try to leap ahead of the healing process. In other words, healing takes time. To help myself move beyond grief, I decided to talk about my feelings openly. If someone asked me about Mom, I told them the truth.

The outcome of my honesty was surprising. People who had been reserved in the past suddenly opened up to me, and I heard many heartbreaking stories. Our emotional pain bonded us together then, and it continues to bond us together now.

I have great respect for professional, family, and spousal caregivers. Being an Alzheimer's caregiver is hard work. The difference between a "successful" and "unsuccessful" caregiver is often attitude. If I have a negative attitude about caregiving, the result is a negative day. However, if I let myself feel a broad range of emotions, including pain, the result is a successful day. Counselors call this process "going with the pain." My acceptance of pain changed my caregiving. The pain was still there, but it was easier to bear.

AFFIRM YOUR CAREGIVING

Few of the resources I've read talk about the rights of the caregiver. In the past, our society was so focused on the patient's needs that the caregiver's needs fell by the wayside. No more. Researchers and authors like Jo Horne, who wrote *Caregiving: Helping an Aging Loved One,* are writing about caregivers' needs.

The book includes "A Caregiver's Bill of Rights." One point gives the caregiver the right to reject a relative's attempts to manipulate him or her "through guilt, anger, or depression." Blank lines at the bottom of the bill invite readers to add their own points. Readers are advised to go through the list daily.

While "A Caregiver's Bill of Rights" sparked my thinking, it seemed strident to me. Still, the idea of caregivers' rights was a sound one. I decided to affirm my caregiving efforts on paper. With a long-range view in mind, I wrote the following affirmations.

- ➤ I will take good care of myself.
- ➤ I will make "me time" part of every day.
- ➤ I will let myself feel a full range of emotions.
- ➤ I will find comfort in happy memories.
- ➤ I will learn from my mistakes.
- ➤ I will ask others for help.
- ➤ I will give myself time off from caregiving.
- ➤ I will view my caregiving as a whole.
- ➤ I will cherish each moment of life.

As you can see, each affirmation contains the word *will* to signify my resolve. Each affirmation also contains an active verb to get me going. I tried to keep my affirmations simple.

Writing the affirmations was a spiritual experience for me. About all I can do for Mom is pray for her. In the early morning hours, when my husband is still asleep, I think about Mom. I thank God for her life and her love, and I pray for her peaceful death.

RESEARCH UPDATE

Family is the heart of my life, and I draw strength from it. I also draw strength from medical research. Great strides have been made during the last few years, according to the Alzheimer's Association. Researchers are focusing on genetics, drug therapy, early detection, and delaying the onset of the disease.

Alzheimer's is now the fourth largest killer of people in the United States. A recent Alzheimer's Association newsletter, *Advances,* details some of the research in progress. Because identical twins may be symptom-free for years or even permanently, one article asks for volunteers for a Duke University twin study.

Researchers are using genetic testing and brain imaging techniques to track changes in the brain and to spot early signs of Alzheimer's. The newsletter also cites a study by Richard Mayeux, MD, MSR, and his colleagues at Columbia University. Their study showed that postmenopausal women who took estrogens had a lower risk of developing Alzheimer's than women who didn't have estrogen replacement therapy.

Clinical drug trials currently underway are also listed. To learn more about these trials, call the Alzheimer's Association Information and Referral Center at 1-800-272-3900 and ask for the drug fact sheets.

Other Alzheimer's Association research projects are being funded by the Ronald and Nancy Reagan Research Institute. Again, call 1-800-272-3900 to learn more about the Reagan Institute.

Matthew D. Dacy describes the Mayo Clinic Fund for Alzheimer's Research in Honor of President Ronald and Nancy Reagan in a recent issue of *Mayo Magazine*. In response to a matching grant, the clinic has raised more than five million dollars for the fund. Research projects are underway at Mayo Rochester, Mayo Jacksonville, and Mayo Scottsdale. All of the projects have the same goal: to help the patient.

In a recent issue of *Mayo Today*, writer Margaret Koppenhafer describes the research as a "race against time." She discusses some of the steps involved in this race, such as the fact that in 1986 an Alzheimer's Disease Patient Registry was started at Mayo Rochester with funding from the National Institutes of Health. In 1990 the Mayo Alzheimer's Disease Center was started with funds from the National Institutes of Health. Other neuropsychology, neuroimaging, and neurodegenerative disease projects are also underway.

Mayo researchers are also working on applying research findings to patient care via drug treatment trials, community outreach programs, and a Memory Disorder Clinic. Alzheimer's research is bringing Mayo sites, scientists, and practicing physicians together in one concentrated effort.

Other researchers, including Mario F. Mendez, MD, PhD, are tailoring existing tests to Alzheimer's patients. Mendez and his colleagues detail their work in "Development of Scoring Criteria for the Clock Drawing Task in Alzheimer's Disease."

They ask: Can the Clock Drawing Interpretation Scale be used with probable Alzheimer's patients? Forty-six patients with probable Alzheimer's participated in the study. These patients were compared with twenty-six healthy elderly people, the controls. The clock drawing test and other neuropsychological tests were administered to all study participants.

Despite the Alzheimer's patients' problems with visual perception, the researchers feel that the clock drawing test may be used with demented patients. A "Clock Drawing Interpretation Scale" was developed by the researchers to go along with the original test. This is just one example of how researchers are adapting to patient needs.

EACH PATIENT IS UNIQUE

When you know one patient, you don't know them all. Each is unique. This book summarizes the latest caregiving research and the problems that caregivers face. I have used my mother as an example to make the research come alive.

The book brings my mother's story to a close. Writing it brought back many childhood memories. Before the onset of dementia, my mother was an intelligent, vital, and vibrant woman. Pictures of Mom pass through my mind like movie film rolling backwards.

I see her at the kitchen sink, washing dishes in sudsy water, and singing Broadway songs at the top of her lungs. She has brought home a gyroscope from the Sperry plant, where she is an assembly line worker, and spins it on the table top to show us how it works. Hurrying to get ready for church, she pushes her hair behind her ears, and dons a black picture hat.

Her face is filled with pride when I graduate from college. With a sparkle in her eyes, she gives Dad a cake that reads "Happy 50th Anniversary Darling." More recently, I see Mom sitting in a wingback chair, wearing a flowered blouse, her hair newly coifed, and holding two wiggling babies on her lap.

These pictures fade to a picture of Mom today, lying in a recliner and staring vacantly into space. She is a broken woman. I can't alter the ravages of time and disease, but I can make sure that she gets good care.

Caregiving is a personal journey, and the days are filled

with discoveries. Some days go better than others. When the days are dark, we may be guided by the beacons of research. When the days are long, we may be refreshed by happy memories. When the days are gone, we will know we have done our best.

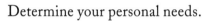

What Can You Do?

Determine your personal needs.

Make a self-care plan.

Avoid the martyr trap.

Get regular check-ups.

Every so often do an "interior clean-up."

Figure out how to be more efficient.

Pace yourself.

Make "me time" a part of every day.

Become a steward of the patient's values.

Learn more about dementia.

Let yourself grow from pain.

Affirm your caregiving.

Revise your self-care plan regularly.

Remember, the caregiving you do isn't a job; it is sacred to life itself.

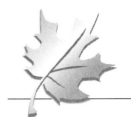

Appendix A
Grief Triggers
Log Form

Date	Incident	Why am I grieving?

Date	Incident	Why am I grieving?

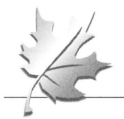

Loss History
Graph Form

midlife

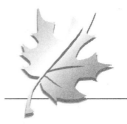

Appendix C

Pleasurable Activities Form

I really enjoy:

_____

_____

_____

_____

_____

_____

_____

_____

I would like to try:

_____

_____

_____

_____

_____

_____

_____

_____

_____

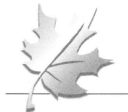

"I Need" Planning Form

Think about the future. Are there things you need to do for yourself in order to get there? List your needs here on the blank lines. Check them off as you do them.

❏ _____

❏ _____

❏ _____

❏ _____

❏ _____

❏ _____

❏ _____

❏ _____

❏ _____

❏ _____

❏ _____

❏ _____

❏ _____

❏ _____

❏ _____

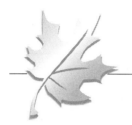

Resources

Abbe, Mary. "Portrait of the Artist as an Old Man," *Minneapolis Star Tribune*, February 4, 1996, pp. 1F, 5F.

"A Little Planning Makes Eating Right a Piece of Cake," in *Day By Day: Caring For Patients With Alzheimer's* (newsletter), Fall 1993, p. 4.

"Always Keep a Helping Hand Within Easy Reach," in *Day By Day: Caring For Patients With Alzheimer's* (newsletter), Fall 1993, p. 3.

Alzheimer's Association. *Advances* (research newsletter), Spring 1997, vol. 2, no. 1.

Alzheimer's Association. *Alzheimer's Disease: Services You May Need* (pamphlet).

Alzheimer's Association. "Distance Complicates Caregiving," *Alzheimer's Association National Newsletter*, Fall 1996, pp. 1, 7.

Alzheimer's Association. "Combativeness," *Third Annual Mayo Alzheimer's Disease Center Conference for Families* (conference program), Rochester, Minnesota, November 1996.

Alzheimer's Association. "Families Find Comfort in Hospice Care," *Alzheimer's Association National Newsletter*, Spring 1996, pp. 1, 7.

Alzheimer's Association. *Legal Considerations for Alzheimer's Patients* (brochure). Chicago: Alzheimer's Association, 1991.

Alzheimer's Association. "Making Home a Safe Place," *Alzheimer's Association National Newsletter*, Fall 1996, p. 3.

Alzheimer's Association. "When It's Time to Consider Other Options," in *Day By Day: Caring For Patients With Alzheimer's* (newsletter), Fall 1993, p. 3.

"Alzheimer's: The Long Goodbye," CNN television special, February 9, 1996.

American Association of Retired Persons. *Depression Later in Life* (brochure), 1993, pp. 1–3.

Anderson, A., et al. "Unsung Heroes," *Home Healthcare Nurse*, November–December 1995, pp. 9–15.

Ballard, Edna L., MSW, ACSW, and Poer, Cornelia M., BA. *Sexuality and the Alzheimer's Patient*. Durham, NC: Duke University, 1993, pp. 6–7, 10, 14–15, 35–37, 54.

Batchelder, Kay, family caregiver interview in February 1997.

Berger, Lisa. *Feathering Your Nest: The Retirement Planner*. New York: Workman Publishing, 1993, pp. 54, 101–103, 256, 444.

Bergman-Evans, Brenda F., RNC, PhD, "Alzheimer's and Related Disorders: Loneliness, Depression, and Social Support of Spousal Caregivers," *Journal Of Gerontological Nursing*, March 1994, pp. 6–16.

Boyd, Malcom. "Weeding Out the Blues," *Modern Maturity*, December 1993–January 1994, p. 72.

Boykin, Anne, PhD, RN, and Winland-Brown, Jill, EdD, RN. "The Dark Side of Caring: Challenges of

Caregiving," *Journal of Gerontological Nursing,* May 1995, pp. 13–18.

Bozarth-Campbell, Alla, PhD. *Life Is Goodbye, Life Is Hello: Grieving Well Through All Kinds of Loss.* Minneapolis: CompCare Publications, 1986, p. 5, 53, 54, 65.

Bozzola, Fernando G., MD, et al. "Personality Changes in Alzheimer's Disease," *Archives of Neurology,* March 1992, pp. 297–300.

Braiker, Harriet B., PhD. *Getting Up When You're Feeling Down.* New York: Pocket Books, 1988, pp. 263–264.

Buckman, Dr. Robert. *"I Don't Know What to Say": How to Help and Support Someone Who Is Dying.* Boston: Little, Brown, 1989, p. 141.

Budnick, Herbert N., PhD. *Heart to Heart: A Guide to the Psychological Aspects of Heart Disease.* Santa Fe: Health Press, pp. 49-51.

Burns, Alistair, et al. "Psychiatric Phenomena in Alzheimer's Disease: Disorders of Thought Content," *British Journal of Psychiatry,* July 1990, p. 72.

Burns, David D., MD. *Feeling Good: The New Mood Therapy.* New York: William Morrow and Company, Inc. 1980, pp. 364–365.

Cammer, Leonard, MD. *Up from Depression.* New York: Simon & Schuster, 1969, pp. 3–15.

Centers for Disease Control. "Alzheimer's Hits Elderly Whites Most Often," *American Medical News,* April 9, 1996, p. 28.

Chaplin, James P., PhD. *Dictionary of Psychology.* New York: Dell Publishing, 1985, p. 203.

Chatterjee, Anjan, MD, et al. "Personality Changes in Alzheimer's Disease," *Archives of Neurology*, May 1992, pp. 486–491.

Chicago Tribune. "Is Forgetting A Danger Sign?" reprinted in *The Arizona Republic*, March 16, 1997, p. A2.

Clifford, Dennis. *The Power of Attorney Book*. New York: Nolo Books, 1990, section 1, pp. 2–33.

Connell, Cathleen M., PhD, et al. "Increasing Coordination of the Dementia Service Delivery Network: Planning for the Community Outreach Education Program," *Gerontologist*, October 1994, pp. 700–706.

Dacy, Matthew D. "Alzheimer's Disease: Matching Grant Opens New Research Horizons," *Mayo Magazine*, Spring/Summer 1997, pp. 40–41.

David, Charles. "The Resurrection-of-the-Dead Syndrome," *American Journal of Psychotherapy*, January 1980, pp. 119–126.

Davies, Helen D., MS, RNCS, et al. "Til Death Do Us Part: Intimacy and Sexuality in the Marriages of Alzheimer's Patients," *Journal of Psychological Nursing and Mental Health Services*, November 1992, pp. 5–10.

Devanand, D. P., MD, et al. "Behavioral Syndromes in Alzheimer's Disease," *International Psychogeriatrics*, Supplement 1, 1992, pp. 161, 163–165, 176–177.

Dubinsky, Richard M., MD, et al. "Driving in Alzheimer's Disease," *Journal of the American Geriatric Society*, November 1992, pp. 1112–1116.

Enlow, Pamela N., MSN, RN. "Coping with Anticipatory Grief," *Journal of Gerontological Nursing*, July 1989, pp. 36–37.

Ernst, Richard L., and Hay, Joel W., PhD. "The U.S. Economic and Social Costs of Alzheimer's Disease Revisited," *American Journal of Public Health*, August 1994, pp. 1261–1264.

Eskes, David. "Holding Back the Sunset," *Phoenix Magazine*, October 1965, pp. 60–66.

"Families of Alzheimer's Patients Need Your Help Too," *American Medical News*, March 17, 1997, p. 17.

Fulton, Robert, PhD, and Bendiksen, Robert, PhD. *Death & Identity*. Philadelphia: The Charles Press, Publishers, Inc., 1994, pp. 168–169, 172–173.

Gallienne, Robert L., BA, RN, ND, et al. "Alzheimer's Caregivers: Psychosocial Support via Computer Networks," *Journal of Gerontological Nursing*, December 1993, pp. 15–22.

Gerdner, Linda A., MA, RN, and Buckwalter, Kathleen C., PhD, RN, FAAN. "A Nursing Challenge: Assessment and Management of Agitation in Alzheimer's Patients," *Journal of Gerontological Nursing*, April 1994, pp. 11–20.

Goldsmith, Seth B. *Choosing a Nursing Home*. New York: Prentice Hall Press, 1990, pp. 2–5, 60–62, 157–167.

Gregor, Joan, RN, professional caregiver, phone interview, February 1997.

Hall, Geri Richards, MA, RN, CS, et al. "Caring for People with Alzheimer's Disease Using the Conceptual Model of Progressively Lowered Stress in a Clinical Setting," *Nursing Clinics of North America*, March 1994, pp. 129–141.

Hall, Geri Richards, MA, RN, CS, et al., "Standardized Care Plan: Managing Patients at Home," *Journal of Gerontological Nursing*, January 1995, pp. 37–47.

Hall, R. R. "Standardized Care Plan: Managing Alzheimer's Patients at Home," *Journal of Gerontological Nursing*, January 1995, pp. 37–47.

Hamilton, Andrea. "Living with Alzheimer's," *Rochester Post-Bulletin*, June 19, 1995, p. 1C.

Heathman, Joanne, RN, CS, GNP. "Late-Stage Needs and Issues in Dementia." *Third Annual Mayo Alzheimer's Disease Center Conference for Families* (conference program), Rochester, Minnesota, November 1996.

Hendren, John. "In 'Snoezelin Room' Alzheimer's Takes a Nap," *Rochester Post-Bulletin*, November 27, 1996, p. 1D.

Hodgson, Harriet. *Alzheimer's: Finding the Words*. Minneapolis: Chronimed Publishing, 1995, p. IV.

Hoffman, Catherine, ScD, et al. "Persons with Chronic Conditions: Their Prevalence and Costs," *Journal of the American Medical Association* (JAMA), November 13, 1996, pp. 1473–1479.

Hoffman, Robert, family caregiver, phone interview on July 14, 1997.

Horne, Jo. *Caregiving: Helping an Aging Loved One*. Glenview, IL: Scott, Foresman and Company, 1985, pp. 51, 94–99, 136, 249–250.

Horne, Jo. *The Nursing Home Handbook: A Guide for Families*. Glenview, IL: Scott, Foresman and Company, 1989, pp. 4, 32–39.

Hurly, A. C. "Reaching Consensus: The Process of Recommending Treatment Decisions for Alzheimer's Patients," *Advances in Nursing Science*, December 1995, pp. 33–43.

James, John W., and Cherry, Frank. *The Grief Recovery Handbook: A Step-by-Step Program for Moving Beyond Loss*. New York: Harper & Row, pp. 91–94.

Jeste, Dilip V., MD, et al. "Cognitive Deficits of Patients with Alzheimer's Disease With and Without Delusions," *American Journal of Psychiatry*, February 1992, pp. 184–189.

Karr, Katherine L. *Promises to Keep: The Family's Role in Nursing Home Care*. Buffalo, NY: Prometheus Books, 1991, pp. 13–14, 83, 99.

Kerr, Rita Butchko. "Meanings Adult Daughters Attach to a Parent's Death," *Western Journal of Nursing Research*, vol. 16, no. 4, 1994, pp. 347–365.

Kimmelman, Michael. "Willem de Kooning Dies at 92; Reshaped U.S. Art," *The New York Times*, March 20, 1997, pp. A1, A16.

Konek, Carol Wolfe. *Daddyboy: A Memoir*. St. Paul: Graywolf Press, 1991, pp. 36, 48, 74, 120–121.

Koppenhafer, Margaret. "A Race Against Time," *Mayo Today*, November 1995, pp. 24–25.

Kubler-Ross, Elisabeth. *On Death and Dying*. New York: Collier Books, 1969, p. 4.

Larkin, Marilynn. *When Someone You Love Has Alzheimer's*. New York: Dell Publishing, 1994, pp. 12, 184–200, 224.

Larson, Eric B., MD, MPH. "Alzheimer's Disease in the Community," *Journal of the American Medical Association* (JAMA), November 10, 1996, pp. 2591–2592.

Leon, Joel, MD. "The 1990–1991 National Survey of Special Care Units in Nursing Homes," *Alzheimer's Disease & Associated Disorders*, Supplement 1, 1994, pp. 572–586.

Lockert, Anya. "Finding Comfort in Rituals," *Rochester Post-Bulletin*, October 26, 1996, p. 9C.

Lopez, Oscar L., MD. "Alzheimer's Disease and Depression: Neuropsychological Impairment and Progression of Illness," *American Journal of Psychiatry*, July 1990, pp. 855–860.

Mace, Nancy L. and Rabins, Peter V., MD. *The 36-Hour Day*. New York: Warner Books, 1981, pp. 242–243, 314–315.

Majeski, Tom. "Many Get Blue from the Lack of White Light," *Minneapolis Star Tribune*, January 2, 1993, p. 1E.

Mann, U. M., et al. "Rapidly Progressing Alzheimer's Disease," *The Lancet*, September 30, 1989, p. 799.

"Marketing That Pays," *Assisted Living Today*, Summer 1994, p. 20.

Mayo Foundation for Medical Education and Research. "Alzheimer's Disease: Living with a 'Long Goodbye'" (supplement to *Mayo Clinic Health Letter*), October 1996, pp.1–8.

Mayo Foundation for Medical Education and Research. "Sexuality and Aging" (supplement to *Mayo Clinic Health Letter*), February 1993, pp. 1–8.

McCabe, Barbara W., et al. "Availability and Utilization of Services by Alzheimer's Disease Caregivers," *Journal of Gerontological Nursing*, January 1995, pp. 14–22.

McIlrath, Sharon. "Medigap Under Fire: Can It Be Fixed or Should It Be Ditched?" *American Medical News*, March 3, 1997, pp. 3, 34.

Mehr, David R., MD, MS, and Fries, Brant E., PhD. "Resource Use on Alzheimer's Special Care Units," *The Gerontologist*, April 1995, pp. 179–184.

Mendez, Mario F., MD, PhD, et al. "Development of Scoring Criteria for the Clock Drawing Task in Alzheimer's Disease," *American Geriatrics Society*, November 1992, pp. 1095–1099.

Menninger, Karl, MD. "A Declaration of Probable Needs," *Menninger Perspective*, November 1, 1996, pp. 26–29.

Moffatt, Bettyclare. *Soulwork: Clearing the Mind, Opening the Heart, Replenishing the Spirit*. Berkeley: Wildcat Canyon Press, pp. 35–36, 140–143, 177–181.

Myers, Edward. *When Parents Die: A Guide for Adults*. New York: Penguin Books, 1986, pp. 80–105.

Neal, Leslie Jean, "The Home Care Client with Alzheimer's Disease: Part I: Assessment Tools for Activities of Daily Living," *Home Healthcare Nurse*, March 1996, pp. 175–178.

Oestreich, Ken. "Make Sure Your Benefits Will Be There," *Rochester Post-Bulletin*, February 28, 1997, p. 3D.

Osmont, Kelly. *More Than Surviving*. Omaha, NE: Centering Corporation, 1990, p. 56.

Parke-Davis. "Always Keep a Helping Hand Within Easy Reach." *Day by Day: Caring for Patients with Alzheimer's,* Fall 1993, p. 3.

Parke-Davis. *Caring for the Caregiver: A Guide To Living With Alzheimer's Disease.* Warner-Lambert Company, 1994, pp. 13–25.

"Patient with Alzheimer's Not Responsible for Injuring Nurse," *American Medical News,* March 11, 1996, p. 22.

Perrone, Janice. "Depression Research Strides May Help Prevent Suicides," *American Medical News,* March 10, 1997, pp. 10–11.

Peterson, Karen S. "Helping Hands for Caregivers," *USA Today,* March 18, 1997, p. 4D.

Peterson, Karen S. "More Spend Time Caring for Elders," *USA Today,* March 18, 1997, p. 1D.

Petrie, Mary, RN, Program Administrator, Alzheimer's Unit, University Good Samaritan Health Care Center, Minneapolis, MN, Speaker, Alzheimer's Association Southern Regional Conference, July 30, 1996.

Pieper, Hanns G. *The Nursing Home Primer: A Comprehensive Guide to Nursing Homes and Other Long-Term Care Options.* White Hall, VA: Betterway Publications, Inc., 1989, pp. 39–52, 58, 61–64.

Rando, Therese A. *Loss & Anticipatory Grief.* New York: Lexington Books, 1986, pp. 1–79.

Rando, Therese A. "Anticipatory Grief: The Term Is a Misnomer but the Phenomenon Exists," *Journal of Palliative Care,* February 1988, pp. 70–73.

Rice, Dorothy P. et al. "The Economic Burden of Alzheimer's Disease Care," *Health Affairs*, Summer 1993, pp. 164–176.

Richards, Geri Hall, MA, RN, CS. "Caring for People with Alzheimer's Disease Using the Conceptual Model of Progressively Lowered Stress Threshold in the Clinical Setting," *Nursing Clinics of North America*, March 1994, pp. 129–133.

Richter, Judith M., et al. "Communicating with Persons with Alzheimer's Disease: Experiences of Family and Formal Caregivers," *Archives of Psychiatric Nursing*, October 1995, pp. 279–285.

Rinard, Peggy. "Close-Up Look at the Wonders of the Brain," *University of Minnesota Medical Bulletin*, Fall 1996, p. 6.

Ripich, D. N., et al. "Alzheimer's Disease Caregivers: The FOCUSED Program." *Geriatric Nursing*, January–February 1995, pp. 15–19.

Rosen, Eliott. *Families Facing Death*. Lexington, MA: D. C. Heath and Company, 1990, p. 95.

Sambandham, Mary, MSN, RN, and Schirm, Victoria, PhD, RN. "Music as a Nursing Intervention for Residents with Alzheimer's Disease in Long-Term Care," *Geriatric Nursing*, March-April 1995, pp. 79–83.

Sandlin, Nina, compiler. "What's the Deal with All This Free Medicine?" *American Medical News*, March 17, 1997, p. 23.

Shelton, Deborah L. "More Geriatrics Training Needed as Population Ages," *American Medical News*, November 11, 1996, p. 5.

Shockman, Luke. "Alzheimer's: First, They Have to Understand It," *Rochester Post-Bulletin*, May 25, 1996, p. 6B.

Shockman, Luke. "Alzheimer's: Losing Time," *Rochester Post-Bulletin*, May 25, 1996, p. 1B.

Shockman, Luke. "Caring for the Caregiver," *Rochester Post-Bulletin*, October 28, 1996, p. 1D.

Smith, Dorothy B., RN, MS, CETN, OCN, FAAN. "Staffing and Managing Special Care Units for Alzheimer's Patients," *Geriatric Nursing*, May–June 1995, pp. 124–127.

"Society Pays Cost for Undertreatment of Depression," *American Medical News*, January 27, 1997, p. 10.

Steele, Cynthia, RN, MPH, et al. "Psychiatric Symptoms in Nursing Home Placement of Patients with Alzheimer's Disease," *American Journal of Psychiatry*, August 1990, pp. 1049–1151.

Tangalos, Eric, MD. "Make a Resolution You Can Be Healthier With," *Rochester Post-Bulletin*, December 31, 1996, p. 8A.

Tanzer, Sheila Harvey. "In the Wake of Loss," *Dartmouth Magazine*, Fall 1995, pp. 42–45.

Theut, Susan K., MD, MPH, et al. "Caregiver's Anticipatory Grief in Dementia: A Pilot Study," *International Journal of Aging and Development*, vol. 33, 1992, pp. 113–118.

U.S. Department of Health and Human Services. *Guide for Choosing a Nursing Home*. Baltimore: U.S. Government Printing Office, 1994, pp. 1–18.

U.S. Department of Health and Human Services. *Guide to Health Insurance for People with Medicare.* Baltimore: U.S. Government Printing Office, 1996, pp. 2–10.

U.S. Department of Health and Human Services. *Your Medicare Handbook.* Baltimore: U.S. Government Printing Office, 1996, pp. 11–17.

Viorst, Judith. *Necessary Losses.* New York: Fawcett Gold Medal, 1986, p. 248–261.

Welch, Deborah, RN, MSN. "Anticipatory Grief Reactions in Family Members of Adult Patients," *Issues in Mental Health Nursing,* vol. 4, no. 2, 1982, pp. 148–158.

Welch, H. Gilbert, MD, MPH, et al. "The Cost of Institutional Care in Alzheimer's Disease: Nursing Home and Hospital Use in a Prospective Cohort," *Journal of the American Geriatric Society,* March 1992, pp. 221–224.

"When Depression Turns Deadly," *Modern Maturity,* December 1993–January 1994, p. 74.

"When It's Time to Consider Options," *Day By Day: Caring For Patients With Alzheimer's,* (newsletter), Fall 1993, p. 3.

Woititz, Janet Geringer, EdD. *Adult Children of Alcoholics.* No City: Health Communications, 1983, pp. 103–105.

Wolfe, Warren. "Helping Dad by Helping Themselves," *Minneapolis Star Tribune,* November 19, 1995, p. 1B.

Wright, Lore K. "Alzheimer's Disease Afflicted Spouses Who Remain at Home: Can Human Dialectics Explain the Findings?" *Social Science and Medicine,* April 1994, pp. 1037–1046.

Zandi, Taher, Dr. "Understanding Difficult Behaviors of Nursing Home Residents: A Prerequisite for Sensitive Clinical Assessment and Care," *Alzheimer's Disease and Associated Disorders,* Supplement 1, 1994, pp. 345-354.

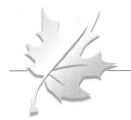

Index

About the Author

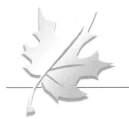

Harriet Hodgson has been a nonfiction writer for more than twenty-one years. She has a BS degree in Early Childhood Education, with honors, from Wheelock College in Boston, and an MA in Art Education from the University of Minnesota in Minneapolis. After twelve years of teaching, she decided to change careers and turned to writing.

An experienced writer, Hodgson is the author of nineteen books for parents and children, plus many newspaper and magazine articles. She is a contributing writer for *The Mayo Clinic Complete Book of Pregnancy & Baby's First Year.* She has also written four Mayo Clinic books to help pediatric patients to prepare for heart surgery.

Hodgson was both narrator and writer for *Parent Talk,* broadcast on Minnesota Public Radio. A frequent radio and television guest, she has appeared on 105 radio talk shows, including CBS and WCCO Radio. She has also appeared on many TV shows including KSTP and CNN, and is a freelance special features writer for the *Rochester Post-Bulletin.*

The mother of two grown daughters, and the proud grandmother of twins, Hodgson lives in Rochester, Minnesota with her husband, John.

ALSO BY HARRIET HODGSON

Alzheimer's: Finding the Words

A Communication Guide for Those Who Care

"[her] ability to probe beneath the surface of behaviors makes this an especially valuable book for formal and informal caregivers.... Hodgson's direct and folksy writing style makes for quick and easy reading."
—*American Journal of Alzheimer's Disease*

Includes a short-term memory questionnaire and insightful interviews with physicians, caregivers, family members, and patients. 1-56561-071-7, $10.95

ORDER BY MAIL

Chronimed Publishing
P.O. Box 59032, Minneapolis, MN 55459-0032
Send check or money order—no cash or C.O.D.s. Please add $3.00 to this order to cover postage and handling. Minnesota residents add 6.5% sales tax. Prices and availability are subject to change without notice.

Name _____

Address _____

City _____

State _____ ZIP _____

Phone _____

ORDER BY PHONE—1-800-848-2793

(612-513-6475 in the Mpls/St. Paul metro area) Please have your credit card ready. Allow 4 to 6 weeks for delivery. Quantity discounts available upon request. Prices and availability subject to change without notice.